ATTENTION DEFICIT

How Technology Has Hijacked Our Ability to Concentrate

Stuart A. Kallen

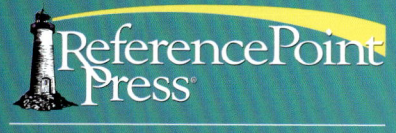

San Diego, CA

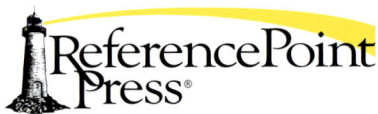

© 2023 ReferencePoint Press, Inc.
Printed in the United States

For more information, contact:
ReferencePoint Press, Inc.
PO Box 27779
San Diego, CA 92198
www.ReferencePointPress.com

ALL RIGHTS RESERVED.
No part of this work covered by the copyright hereon may be reproduced or used in any form or by any means—graphic, electronic, or mechanical, including photocopying, recording, taping, web distribution, or information storage retrieval systems—without the written permission of the publisher.

LIBRARY OF CONGRESS CATALOGING-IN-PUBLICATION DATA

Names: Kallen, Stuart A., 1955- author.
Title: Attention deficit : how technology has hijacked our ability to concentrate / by Stuart A. Kallen.
Description: San Diego, CA : ReferencePoint Press, Inc., 2023. | Includes bibliographical references and index.
Identifiers: LCCN 2022009599 (print) | LCCN 2022009600 (ebook) | ISBN 9781678204549 (library binding) | ISBN 9781678204556 (ebook)
Subjects: LCSH: Cell phones--Psychological aspects. | Internet addiction. | Attention. | Distraction (Psychology)
Classification: LCC RC569.5.I54 K35 2023 (print) | LCC RC569.5.I54 (ebook) | DDC 616.85/84--dc23/eng/20220405
LC record available at https://lccn.loc.gov/2022009599
LC ebook record available at https://lccn.loc.gov/2022009600

CONTENTS

Introduction   4
Smartphones and Ancient Brains

Chapter One   8
Digitally Connected 24/7

Chapter Two   20
Rearranging the Brain

Chapter Three   32
The Myth and Reality of Multitasking

Chapter Four   43
Time for a Digital Detox?

Source Notes	54
Tips for Reducing Digital Distractions	58
For Further Research	59
Index	61
Picture Credits	64
About the Author	64

INTRODUCTION

Smartphones and Ancient Brains

The world is populated by distracted students, distracted parents, and distracted workers. Some of the most popular YouTube videos show distracted pedestrians walking into poles and falling into holes as they stare at their smartphones. While the videos might elicit a chuckle, distracted walking is dangerous. Referring to this problem, the American Academy of Orthopaedic Surgeons warns, "Today, more and more people are falling down stairs, tripping over curbs and other streetscapes and, in many instances, stepping into traffic, causing cuts, bruises, sprains, and fractures."[1]

While thousands wind up in emergency rooms every year due to distracted walking, the problem of distracted driving is even more serious. The National Safety Council says 1.6 million car crashes every year, or one in four, are caused by people using cell phones while driving. Around 390,000 people are injured annually in distracted driving incidents, and more than 3,000 are killed.

Ever since the first iPhone was introduced in 2007, smartphones have been blamed for causing what might be called a distraction pandemic. According to a 2021 survey by the consumer product review site Reviews.org, Americans over age eighteen check their phones 262 times a day, or about once every 5.5 minutes. The survey found that around half of all Americans spend five to six hours a day on their various mobile devices, and 40 percent look at their phones while driving.

Fifty-four percent said they panic when their cell phone battery runs low on power.

Social media is by far the greatest distraction linked to smartphones because users enjoy the sense of belonging and feel left out if they miss the latest trending post. Following social media, though, can lead to some unhealthy outcomes; users may not feel smart enough, popular enough, wealthy enough, pretty enough, physically fit enough, or cultured enough compared to those who appear to have mastered the medium. Derek Thompson, a staff writer for the *Atlantic*, compares social media sites like Instagram to alcohol: "Delightful but also depressing, a popular experience that blends short-term euphoria with long-term regret, a product that leads to painful and even addictive behavior among a significant minority."[2]

Wired to React

Addictive smartphone behavior can be linked to the way human brains developed over hundreds of millennia to ensure the survival of the species. Humans evolved to be on high alert for dangerous predators and aggressive rivals when searching for food and shelter. Reacting quickly to the noise of a breaking branch or the sight of a fleeting shadow in the forest could mean the difference between life and death.

Warnings that set off primal alarms in the brain are known as bottom-up forces. These forces react to unexpected or dramatic stimuli by sending signals to the brain that instantly break concentration. The thinking processes are overwhelmed by the fight-or-flight response, which prepares the body either to confront danger or flee.

People no longer need to react as often for survival purposes, but smartphones and social media are purposely designed to tap into basic survival systems. Pop-ups, prompts, and notifications send constant signals to the brain and distract people from their routines or tasks at hand. As neuroscientist Adam Gazzaley explains, "Many technological devices use bottom-up stimuli to draw our attention from our goals, like buzzes and vibrations and flashes of light."[3]

A Drain on the Brain

Mindless smartphone use is more than a harmless distraction. Researchers call it a brain drain. A 2017 study by the University of California, Irvine, revealed that it takes an average of twenty-three minutes and fifteen seconds for a person to refocus after a distraction caused by a digital device. In other words, when someone wants to take just thirty seconds to check his or her Instagram feed, he or she is actually going to waste more than twenty minutes. In addition to lowering productivity, the study showed that attention distraction can increase stress and put users in a bad mood. Even if a device is turned off but sitting within reach, it causes distraction.

Living in a world of swipes, clicks, and likes interferes with basic human interactions, according to communications professor Shalini Misra. She writes, "In the presence of a mobile device, there is less eye contact. A person is potentially more likely to miss subtle cues, facial expressions, and changes in the tone of their conversation partner's voice when his or her thoughts are directed to other concerns."[4]

The human brain is far more complex than the newest smartphone or even the entire internet. Neuroscientist Christof Koch of the Allen Institute for Brain Science refers to the brain as "the most complex object in the known universe."[5] Brains contain 86 billion neurons that process information that is sent through a network of hundreds of trillions of connections called synapses. These complex objects, which can store 1 billion bits of data, have allowed people to create astounding art while reshaping the world to ensure survival for billions.

> "Many technological devices use . . . stimuli to draw our attention from our goals, like buzzes and vibrations and flashes of light."[3]
>
> —Adam Gazzaley, neuroscientist

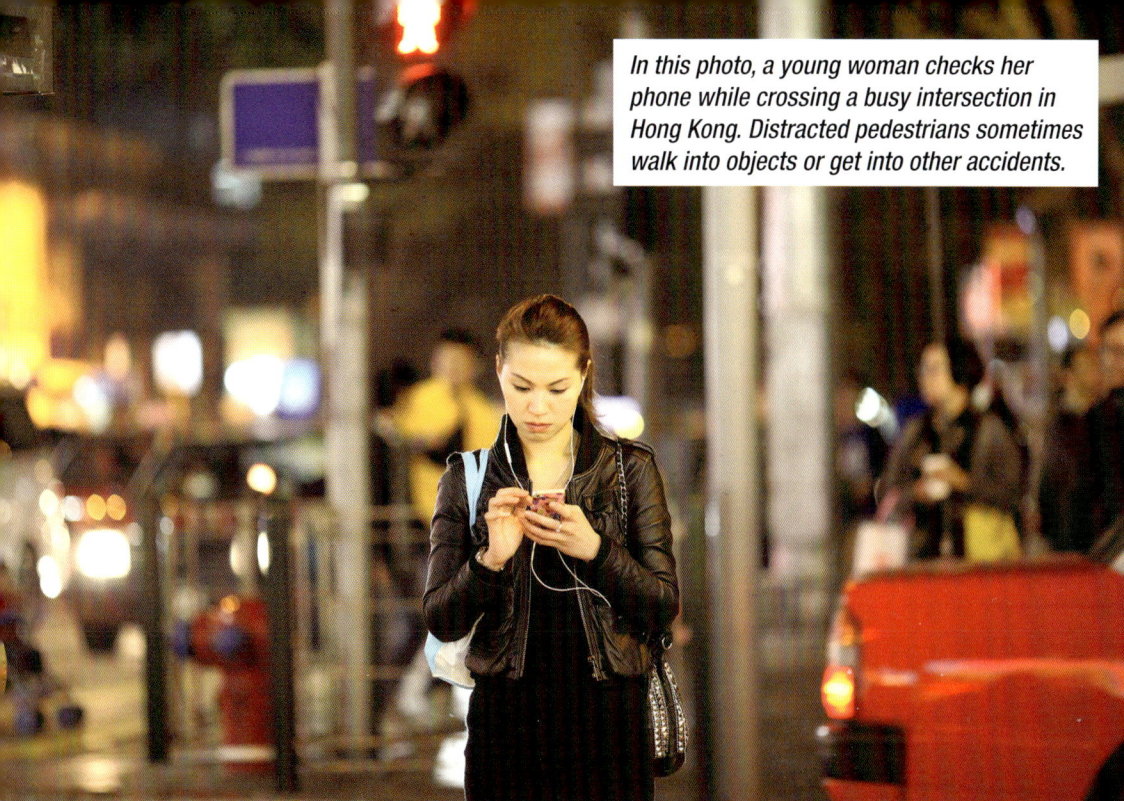

In this photo, a young woman checks her phone while crossing a busy intersection in Hong Kong. Distracted pedestrians sometimes walk into objects or get into other accidents.

People have struggled for centuries to avoid distractions. But the electronic brains that fit in a pocket or purse are making the fight more difficult by the day. Whether the human brain will evolve to deal with distractions of the digital brain remains to be seen. Focusing on the problem and turning off the phone a few hours a day is the first step. Gazzaley remains positive. "By building healthier habits," he says, "we can change our relationship with technology for the better. We're a very adaptive species. I think we'll be OK."[6]

CHAPTER ONE

Digitally Connected 24/7

Justin Rosenstein had had enough of social media. He programmed his laptop to block Reddit. He had an assistant set the parental-control features on his iPhone to prevent him from downloading Facebook. Rosenstein even banned himself from Snapchat; he felt as if the instant messaging app was as addictive as heroin. In 2017, when asked by an interviewer why he took these steps, Rosenstein responded, "Everyone is distracted. All of the time."[7] While many try to limit online distractions, Rosenstein is not a typical social media user; he is the engineer who created the Facebook "Like" button in 2007. Rosenstein earned more than $1 billion from his work at Facebook, but he quit in 2008 because he felt—even at that time—that social media was unhealthy and limited people's ability to focus.

Rosenstein went on to become a leading critic of the attention economy. This term is used to describe an economic model used by Facebook, Instagram, Snapchat, TikTok, YouTube, and other tech companies that build their websites to grab and hold a user's attention. The attention economy gives a new meaning to the term *paying attention*; consumers "pay" for the use of social media sites by constantly focusing on the apps, and companies pay the apps to post ads to give users something to focus on. Rosenstein explained in the 2020 documentary *The Social Dilemma*, "There are all these services on the Internet that we think of as free, but they're not free.

They're paid for by advertisers. Why do advertisers pay those companies? They pay in exchange for showing their ads to us. We're the product. Our attention is the product being sold to advertisers."[8]

> "Everyone is distracted. All of the time."[7]
>
> —Justin Rosenstein, software engineer

Rosenstein, like many Silicon Valley tech executives, sends his children to an elite private school where iPhones, iPads, and even laptops are banned. This is not reality for most people. In 2021, 44 percent of Americans ages eighteen to forty-nine said they were online almost constantly, according to the Pew Research Center. Carolyn Heinrich, a professor of public policy and economics at Vanderbilt University, understands the cost of this behavior: "If someone would have told me I was going to spend 10–12 hours in front of a computer most days to do my job, I would never have chosen my current occupation, but it seems like most jobs these days require constant computer use."[9]

Heinrich says she texts and emails most of her communications, even with colleagues who are sitting in the next office. This constant use of technology has caused her to develop physical problems, including chronic neck and back pain from leaning closer to her monitor. Heinrich also suffers from tendonitis, inflammation of the wrist caused by repetitive use of a computer mouse. And overuse of digital technology can cause more than physical harm. Social media use has been blamed for increasing social isolation and disrupting sleep patterns.

Habit Forming on Purpose

Forty-eight percent of Americans consider themselves addicted to their phones, according to Review.org. David Golumbia, an associate professor of digital studies at Virginia Commonwealth University, is immersed in a culture of digital addiction and distraction. Golumbia says that between one-third and one-half of the students in his classroom are totally checked out. They spend their time staring at a continuous stream of pop-up news alerts,

> "These [smartphones and apps] are designed to steal attention away from anything other than themselves."[10]
>
> —David Golumbia, associate professor of digital studies

instant messages, viral memes, and fifteen-second videos on their phones. Golumbia calls this behavior destructive and overwhelming. And he blames cell phone makers and social media companies for deliberately driving this negative behavior. "These [smartphones and apps] are designed to steal attention away from anything other than themselves,"[10] he says.

Companies at the center of the attention economy—including TikTok, Alphabet (Google and YouTube), and Meta (Facebook and Instagram)—want their apps to be habit forming. Tech executives understand that the more time people spend on their social media platforms, the more money their companies make from advertis-

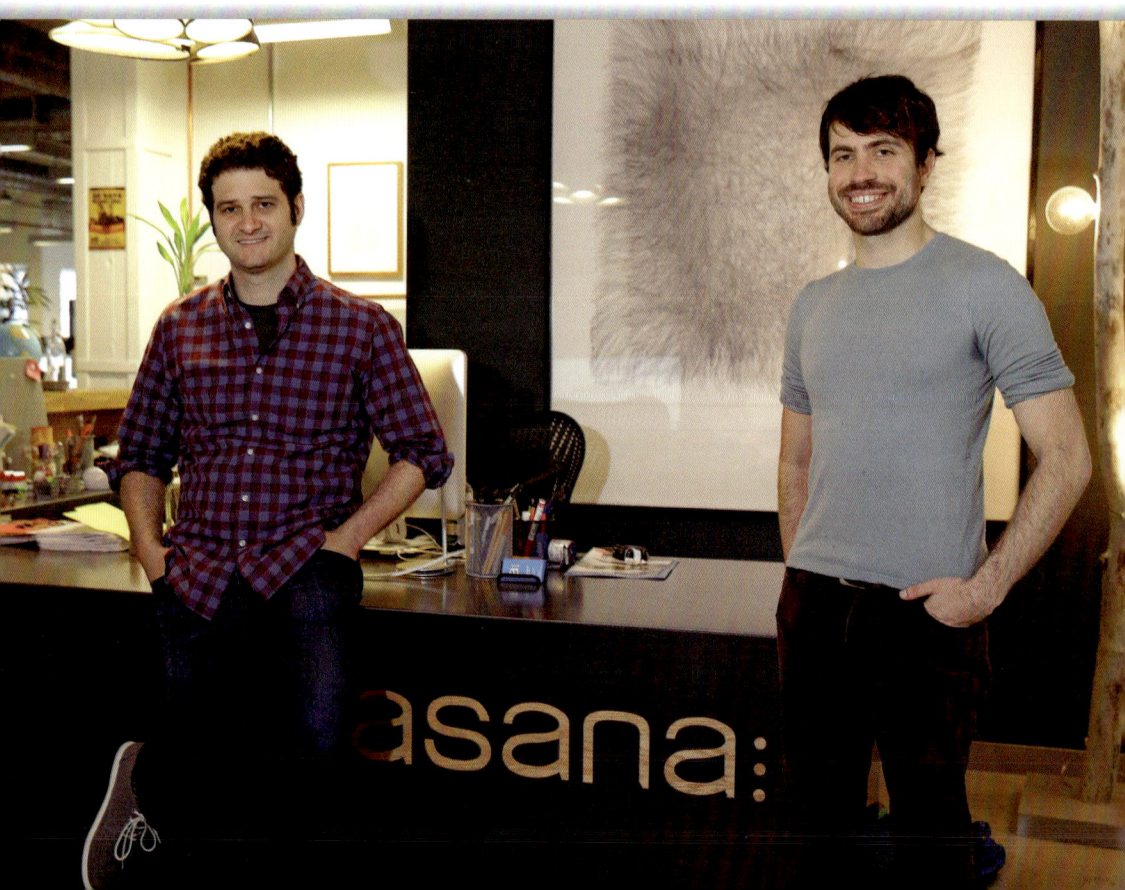

Justin Rosenstein, right, shown in this photo from April 3, 2014, worked for Facebook in the early 2000s and later founded a social media company called Asana before becoming a leading critic of the attention economy.

ing revenue. App developer Peter Mezyk says, "The success of an app is often measured by the extent to which it introduces a new habit."[11]

According to Mezyk, social media companies follow a three-pronged approach to make their apps habit forming. Apps are designed to motivate their use, provide a trigger, and induce an action. Users are often motivated to open an app because of FOMO, or fear of missing out. The knowledge that countless people are posting photos or tweeting about celebrities is too much for some to ignore. This explains why 80 percent of Americans surveyed by Review.org said they open their phones within ten minutes of waking up. Once a user is motivated to open an app, they are triggered to engage with it by a steady stream of clickbait, auto-play videos, and notifications. This hooks users into taking actions that include tapping, clicking, watching, and scrolling for as long as possible.

> "The success of an app is often measured by the extent to which it introduces a new habit."[11]
>
> —Peter Mezyk, app developer

When users are motivated, triggered, and moved to act, the app is deemed a success by the tech company that designed it. But the app distracts users from doing things they might need or want to do. While this might not be a problem in the short term, long-term digital distraction prevents addicted users from living their lives. And it might even undermine their ability to regulate their behavior, which not only impacts these individuals but those around them.

While it is coincidental that the term *user* can be applied to both a person who uses social media and a person who uses drugs, Mezyk sees a link. He says some apps are like helpful supplements such as vitamins, while others are as addictive as painkillers. Apps that work like supplements are not habit forming. They are used for banking, driving directions, translations, or fact-finding. Painkiller apps, however, have a different purpose; they act as sedatives to those suffering from boredom, alienation, and loneliness. Mezyk explains, "Facebook is a good example of a supplement that can quickly transform into a painkiller when you begin to get to the stage where you can't manage without it any longer."[12]

The Person Is the Product

Mezyk believes that apps can be designed to be both beneficial for users and profitable for tech companies. However, this would require the companies to treat social media obsession as a serious problem. This is unlikely because the companies earn billions by keeping people engaged with their screens. This money is generated by artificial intelligence programs that note every action and reaction that users make. The attention that internet users pay to apps is monitored, recorded, and sold to advertisers. Computer scientist Jaron Lanier explains, "[It is] your own behavior and perception that is the product. . . . It's the only possible product. There's nothing else on the table that could possibly be called the product. That's the only thing there is for [tech companies] to make money from."[13]

Tech companies such as Google, Facebook, Twitter, and TikTok compile data on every search, like, comment, posted photo and video, and purchase made by users. The companies also cast a wide net for outside data, grabbing information from apps people use to manage health data, exercise regimens, finances, entertainment choices, and more. Facebook algorithms even categorize users by what are called microexpressions. These tiny details in the position of the mouth, eyes, forehead, and other features are used to determine a user's emotional state in photos and livestreams. Facebook combines this information with other details that supposedly reveal the mind-set of the user. Other data includes the number of exclamation points used in an update and the pattern of likes inserted by a user across the platform. Facebook even uses artificial intelligence to monitor heart rate data from its Instant Heart Rate app.

Artificial intelligence programs comb through this data and come up with fine-grained predictions of what kinds of ads users

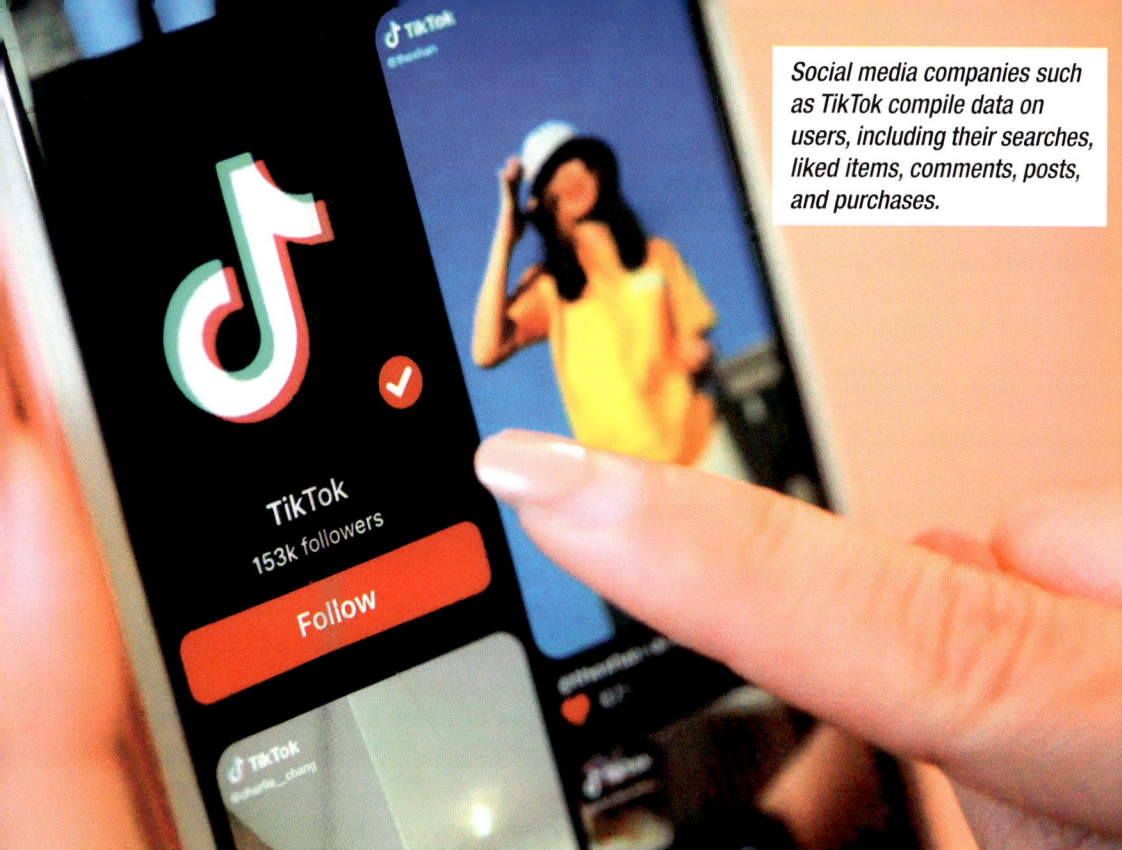

Social media companies such as TikTok compile data on users, including their searches, liked items, comments, posts, and purchases.

will click on and what kinds of products they will buy. This has led to what is called a behavioral prediction industry. Roger McNamee, an early investor in Facebook, says, "Behavioral prediction is about taking uncertainty out of life. Advertising and marketing are all about uncertainty—you never really know who's going to buy your product. Until now. . . . Private corporations have built a corporate surveillance state without our awareness or permission."[14]

Harvard Business School professor Shoshana Zuboff calls this economic model "surveillance capitalism."[15] Zuboff says surveillance capitalism was invented by Google in the early 2000s when it began collecting data about users' search terms, browsing histories, shopping preferences, and other online behavior. As a growing number of users spent more of their time surfing the internet, Google executives realized that they could boost profits by selling private information to advertisers. Zuboff notes, "We thought that we search Google, but now we understand that Google searches us."[16]

A Moral Responsibility

Tristan Harris is a technology ethicist. While working at Google in 2013, he circulated a presentation among employees about the harm that might be caused by addictive smartphones and apps. Harris explained the presentation in the 2020 film *The Social Dilemma*:

> [I said] never before in history have 50 designers—20- to 35-year-old white guys in California—made decisions that would have an impact on two billion people. Two billion people will have thoughts that they didn't intend to have because a designer at Google said, "This is how notifications work on that screen that you wake up to in the morning." And we have a moral responsibility, at Google, for solving this problem. And I sent this presentation to about 15, 20 of my closest colleagues at Google. . . . When I went to work the next day, most of the laptops had the presentation open. Later that day, there was, like, 400 simultaneous viewers. . . . I got e-mails from all around the company. I mean, people in every department saying, "I totally agree." "I see this affecting my kids." "I see this affecting the people around me." "We have to do something about this."

Quoted in Scraps from the Loft, "*The Social Dilemma* (2020)—Transcript," October 3, 2020. https://scrapsfromtheloft.com.

The Google model was embraced by Facebook, Instagram, Twitter, and other social media giants and soon spread across a wide range of sectors, including entertainment, finance, education, and transportation. Zuboff describes how social media companies use every sliver of behavioral data produced by a customer:

> It's not just what you post, it's that you post. It's not just that you make plans to see your friends later. It's whether you say, "I'll see you later" or "I'll see you at 6:45." It's not just that you talk about the things that you have to do today; it's whether you simply rattle them on in a rambling paragraph or list them as bullet points. All of these tiny signals are the behavioral surplus that turns out to have immense predictive value.[17]

Political Distraction

Surveillance capitalism has created some of the wealthiest companies in history. It also provides immense power to those who profit politically by manipulating the thoughts and actions of the digitally distracted. These politicians and supporters are sometimes referred to as conspiracy entrepreneurs. They earn money by knowingly spreading falsehoods about elections, vaccines, political opponents, and other issues.

In 2020 Rudy Giuliani, a personal lawyer for then-president Donald Trump, was one of the nation's most well-known conspiracy entrepreneurs. Giuliani produced YouTube videos that made false claims about widespread voter fraud in the 2020 election that ran on his *Rudy Giuliani's Common Sense* podcast. In addition to promoting wild conspiracy theories, Giuliani earned millions selling a wide range of products, including cigars, gold coins, vitamin supplements, and an untested $596 online fraud-protection system.

Some observers mocked Giuliani's obviously fake claims about the election. But his success as a conspiracy entrepreneur highlights an industry based on trading falsehoods for cash. As reporter Drew Harwell writes:

> Purveyors of falsehoods are often financially rewarded as the audiences for their claims grow. Premium subscriptions, merchandise sales and advertisement revenue form the backbone of the online-influencer economy—and if the audience is buying it, the creators make money, regardless of the facts. . . . Giuliani [is not so much] an ideological crusader but . . . a shrewd marketer eager to monetize his growing fan base, using the kinds of social-media-influencer techniques popular across YouTube, Facebook and Instagram.[18]

According to political scientist Eitan Hersh, there is a huge audience eager for political distraction. Hersh says one-third of Americans admit to spending two or more hours a day paying attention to politics. He depicts a typical day for a person with a digital political obsession: "I refresh my Twitter feed to keep up on the latest political crisis, then toggle over to Facebook to read clickbait news stories, then over to YouTube to see a montage of juicy clips from the latest congressional hearing. I then complain to my family about all the things I don't like that I have seen."[19] Hersh's research shows that these political addicts spend little or no time actually working for change; they simply devote a large portion of their attention to the endless political debates that can be found online.

Working in the Metaverse

The attention drain caused by smartphones and social media is amplified by virtual reality (VR) headsets. While VR has mainly been used in the past by gamers, it is increasingly utilized as a tool for remote workers. One of those workers, Erin McDannald, joins the workforce every day from home when she puts on her Oculus VR headset and motion-capture gloves. The equipment is made by Meta, short for *metaverse*, a term used to describe a wide-ranging, all-inclusive virtual world that is expected to dominate digital life for most people in the future.

McDannald works for an interior design software company called Environments. With the headset on, she feels as if she is walking through the actual office building where Environments was once headquartered. McDannald's avatar in the VR office building works with five other employees who are also represented as avatars. Like real workers, the avatars visit one another's desks, hold meetings, and even celebrate birthdays. McDannald gives a new meaning to being digitally connected when she calls the experience "a merging of our physical and online personas."[20]

While Environments is on the cutting edge of the metaverse, Microsoft founder Bill Gates expects VR to be a part of most workplaces by 2025. He claims, "We're approaching a threshold where the technology begins to truly replicate the experience of

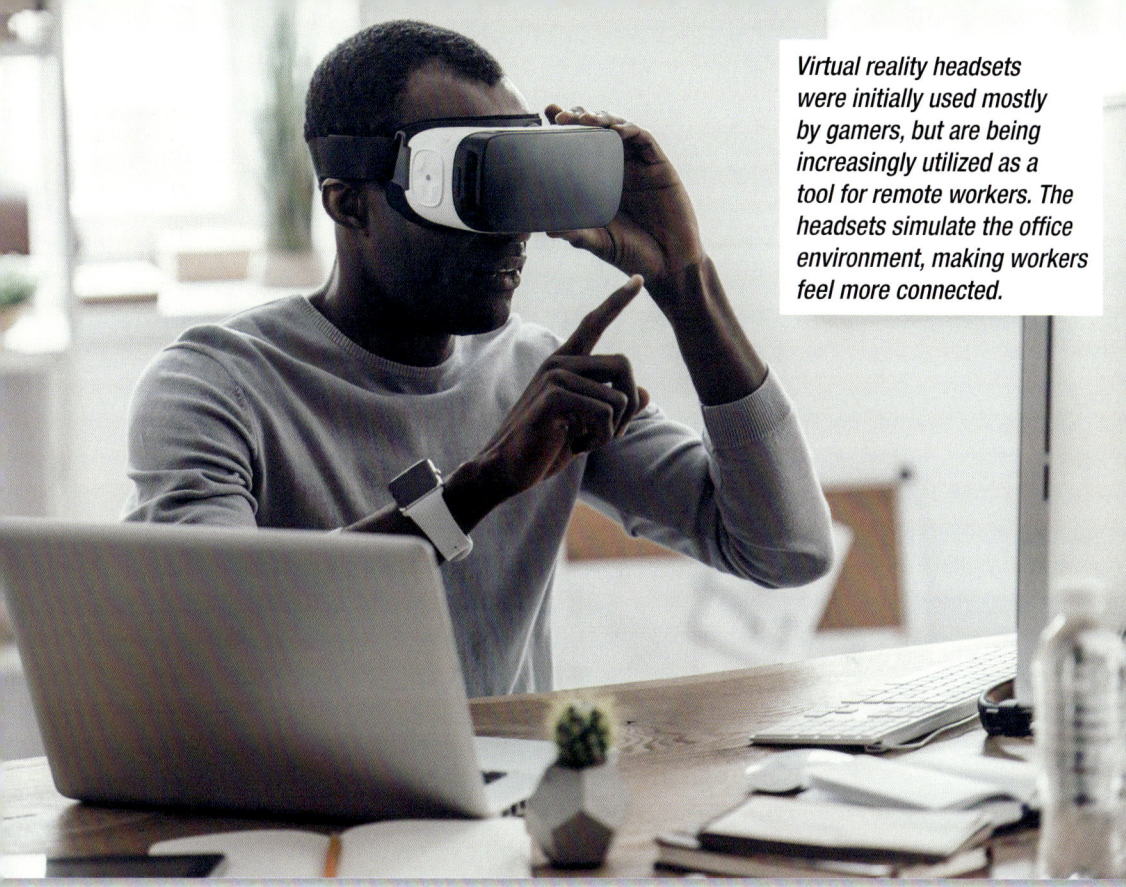

Virtual reality headsets were initially used mostly by gamers, but are being increasingly utilized as a tool for remote workers. The headsets simulate the office environment, making workers feel more connected.

being together in the office."[21] This will benefit companies that will no longer need to buy desks and supplies or rent offices. But some are alarmed at the growing acceptance of the metaverse because it will give tech companies even greater control over people's personal lives.

Meta founder Mark Zuckerberg envisions a day when most people interact with Facebook and Instagram through VR headsets and gloves. These devices track the movement of the eyes and face, allowing software to determine where a user is looking. Eye tracking allows employers to ensure that a worker is paying attention during a meeting and, theoretically, even determine whether the person understands the information being presented. And Meta will be able to collect even more personal data on users in the metaverse. Artificial intelligence programs will gather data on the way the eyes, head, and arms are being moved to further analyze the user's personality, health, and

17

FOMO and Its Consequences

The term *fear of missing out*, or FOMO, came into use in 2004 to describe a phenomenon common on social media sites. The term is often used in a joking or offhanded manner to describe those who constantly update their profile, continually check for likes, and eagerly follow dozens of influencers. However, numerous studies have shown that FOMO is a serious condition that can produce deep feelings of anxiety.

Fear of missing out is caused by influencers and others who bombard social media sites with photos, videos, and stories that paint their lives in the best light. This causes uncertainty in those who wonder whether they are doing enough with their lives. This insecurity can result in compulsive conduct to maintain connections on social media. Those with FOMO might experience negative effects, including poor eating habits, loss of sleep, loss of emotional control, and lack of self-esteem. And the more time users spend on social media, the worse they feel. But few with FOMO are willing to stop. As consumer privacy expert Jeff Tinsley writes, "Many people would rather run a marathon or spend a night in jail than give up their Facebook and Twitter accounts."

Quoted in Adam Gazzaley and Larry D. Rosen, *The Distracted Mind*. Cambridge, MA: MIT Press, 2016, p. 171.

habits. While keeping users overwhelmed with a flood of digital images and sounds, information will be collected to put ads directly in a user's line of vision.

More Distraction Is Coming

Critics insist that the attention economy wastes time and drains energy from the body and brain. And some argue that it also saps the ability of people to live as independent beings in a free society. In 1958 Aldous Huxley, author of the dystopian science-fiction novel *Brave New World*, anticipated this problem. Huxley wrote that defenders of freedom will ultimately be unsuccessful because they "failed to take into account man's almost infinite appetite for distractions." While the internet did not exist at the time, Huxley noted that newspapers, magazines, movies, radios, and television were being "used deliberately . . . for the purpose of preventing people from paying too much attention to the realities of the social and political situation."[22]

While much has changed since Huxley wrote those words, mass media exists for the same reason now as it did back then: to provide a place for advertisers to sell products. In that way Snapchat, TikTok, and Instagram are little different from traditional media. And with bad news dominating the headlines every day, people need distractions from the social and political situation. But it becomes a problem when digital distractions overwhelm the demands of daily life.

There are many, though, who believe that if people understand the forces driving social media, they can limit the distractions in their lives. And this skill will be increasingly necessary, as cofounder of the Center for Humane Technology Tristan Harris says. "The race to keep people's attention isn't going away," he maintains. "Our technology's gonna become more integrated into our lives, not less. The [artificial intelligence programs] are gonna get better at predicting what keeps us on the screen."[23]

> "The race to keep people's attention isn't going away. Our technology's gonna become more integrated into our lives, not less."[23]
>
> —Tristan Harris, technology ethicist

CHAPTER TWO

Rearranging the Brain

In the 1970s intelligence researcher James R. Flynn had a hunch that people throughout the world were getting smarter. Flynn thought this might be due to better nutrition and an increased access to education. He had access to intelligence quotient (IQ) tests given to US soldiers since 1917. These standardized IQ tests were widely used by the military to judge an individual's mental abilities. This allowed the army to assign tasks based on a soldier's intellect.

IQ tests focus on math, memory, reasoning, and verbal ability. Critics say the tests only measure a narrow range of intelligence. But the tests allow researchers to roughly gauge general trends. And Flynn noticed a trend when he compared the early military IQ tests to those that were given to schoolchildren, college students, soldiers, and others in later years. When Flynn began comparing millions of IQ test scores, he discovered that people seemed to be getting more intelligent. In the United States and many other countries, the average IQ score rose by three points every decade, from the low 80s to around 100. This continuous rise in IQ was called the Flynn effect.

In the twenty-first century, the Flynn effect seems to be reversing. In 2009 Flynn discovered that IQs were dropping among teenagers in the United Kingdom. Moreover, while these kids excelled at video gaming, they had difficulty reading or holding a conversation. The reversal of the Flynn effect was also noted in a 2018 Norwegian study of 730,000 IQ tests, which found an average drop of seven IQ points in people born after 1990. Communications researcher Evan Horowitz commented on the study, "People are getting dumber. That's not a judgment; it's a global fact."[24]

Instant Gratification

Few people who use the Internet believe that the ability to instantly access almost all human knowledge is making them dumber. Information is power; it allows people to make personal decisions about their lives in terms of economics, education, personal growth, and more. And the Internet provides data on business, medicine, technology, history, the arts, and more to anyone with a smartphone. But all that information has the ability to overload the brain and change how the memory functions.

> "People are getting dumber. That's not a judgment; it's a global fact."[24]
>
> —Evan Horowitz, communications researcher

According to some experts, people can enter a sort of trance state when they are staring at their screens; their brains are overwhelmed by all the words, pictures, and images. Tech journalist Nicholas Carr explains that this can change how memory functions: "When the brain is overloaded by stimuli, as it usually is when we're peering into a network-connected computer screen, attention splinters, thinking becomes superficial, and memory suffers. We become less reflective and more impulsive. Far from enhancing human intelligence, I argue, the Internet degrades it."[25]

A 2019 study by the journal *World Psychiatry* showed that excessive use of the internet produced "acute and sustained alterations"[26] in the brain. Researchers pointed out that the internet was adopted faster and by more people than any other technology in human history. Billions of people have been searching for information, shopping, consuming entertainment, and socializing online for only the past few decades. These

> "When we're peering into a network-connected computer screen, attention splinters, thinking becomes superficial, and memory suffers."[25]
>
> —Nicholas Carr, tech journalist

rapid changes may have a negative impact on physical brain development and the basic ability to pay attention. According to psychiatry professor Jerome Sarris, "The bombardment of stimuli via the Internet, and the resultant divided attention commonly experienced, presents a range of concerns. I believe that this, along with the increasing #Instagramification of society, has the ability to alter both the structure and functioning of the brain."[27]

Instagramification combines the words *Instagram* with *instant gratification* to define the immediate feelings of happiness Instagram users experience when they see a message that says someone liked their post. The gratification provided by this message and others can be traced to brain chemistry. When people engage in sex, exercise, eating, and some social interactions, the brain releases a pleasure-inducing chemical called dopamine. This chemical is also produced by some drugs. Social media use releases dopamine in the brain of a person whose

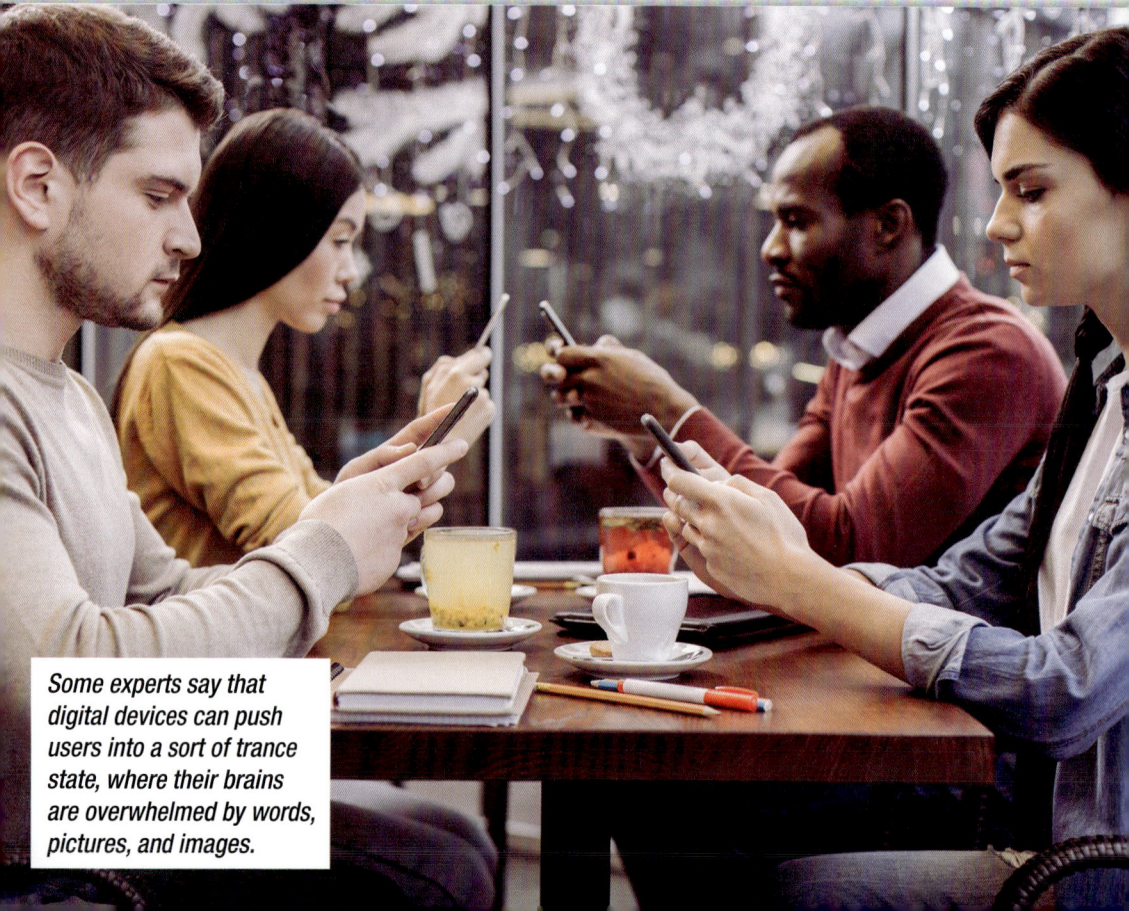

Some experts say that digital devices can push users into a sort of trance state, where their brains are overwhelmed by words, pictures, and images.

news feed is racking up likes, shares, and followers. This causes the user to feel gratified when new notifications pop up. However, the more dopamine people get, the more they want. This anticipation causes people to continually check their phones for notifications. When notifications do not appear, users craving a dose of dopamine can feel anxious and depressed. Rather than put down the phone, they post again and again, hoping their numbers will increase. This can lead to a social media addiction that can be very hard to break.

Internal research conducted by Facebook on its Instagram app in 2021 revealed that the company understands how the cycle of anticipation and reward can affect its users. Facebook found that the Instagram platform left young users feeling addicted—unable to stop themselves from using the app.

While critics often target Instagram, studies show that TikTok can be just as habit forming. Consumer tech journalist John Koetsier compares TikTok to a highly addictive drug, calling the site "digital crack cocaine."[28] Koetsier says his first experience with TikTok had him hooked within a few minutes. Communications professor Julie Albright explains the science behind his obsession: "When you're scrolling . . . sometimes you see a photo or something that's delightful and it catches your attention. And you get that little dopamine hit in the brain . . . in the pleasure center of the brain. So you want to keep scrolling."[29]

> "[With TikTok] you get that little dopamine hit in the brain . . . in the pleasure center of the brain. So you want to keep scrolling."[29]
>
> —Julie Albright, communications professor

As users scroll, they see things they like and things they do not like. Albright compares this to the positive and negative feelings generated by a casino slot machine. According to Albright, "The one thing we know is slot machines are addictive. We know there's a gambling addiction, right? But we don't often talk about how our devices and these [social media] platforms and these apps do have these same addictive qualities baked into them."[30]

The Plastic Brain

In addition to manipulating brain chemistry, overuse of the internet can alter the way the brain functions. These alterations are caused by what is called brain plasticity. The term *plastic* defines anything that is easily shaped or molded. In biology the word *plasticity* is used to describe the makeup of the brain. The billions of nerve cells in the brain, called neurons, are very flexible; they can change their functions to adapt to changing conditions.

Neurons communicate with one another through electric and chemical (electrochemical) signals. These electrochemical signals process a flood of information that pours into the brain through the senses: the eyes, ears, nose, mouth, and nerve endings in the skin. Different parts of the brain are dedicated to each sense. The visual cortex at the back of the brain processes information from the eyes. The audio cortex in the central part of the brain is used to process sounds that enter the ears.

These neural networks have the biological, chemical, and physical ability to reorganize, or rewire themselves, when exposed to new or different information. For example, when individuals lose their sight, they develop a sharpened sense of hearing. This is a result of brain plasticity. The loss of sight causes the visual cortex to change within five days. Some of it falls into disuse, while other parts adapt to better process sounds and tactile information, such as the direction of wind patterns on the skin. These changes help people who lose their sight make their way through the physical world they can no longer see. The brain also modifies itself when it is given new and different information. For example, when a person learns a second language, learns to play the piano, or even takes up juggling, new neural pathways are developed to help him or her perform the new tasks.

The developing brains of young people are more plastic than those of adults. And smartphones can change young brains in many ways. For example, young people can rapidly type on smartphone keyboards with their thumbs. A 2019 study showed

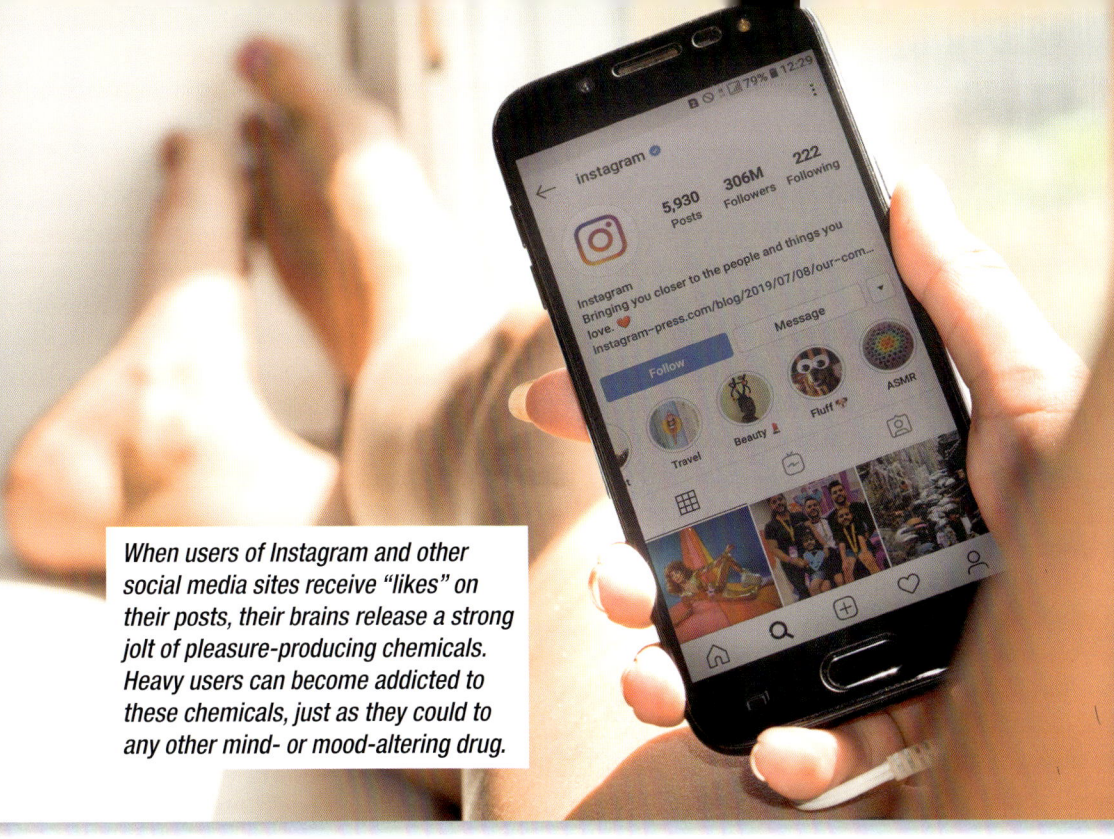

When users of Instagram and other social media sites receive "likes" on their posts, their brains release a strong jolt of pleasure-producing chemicals. Heavy users can become addicted to these chemicals, just as they could to any other mind- or mood-altering drug.

that ten- to nineteen-year-olds type about ten words per minute faster than people in their forties. This is due to changes in the regions of the brain that receive tactile and visual information from the senses. Thanks to brain plasticity, those who type a lot with their thumbs have improved hand-eye coordination, which allows them to effortlessly spell out their thoughts on smartphone keyboards.

Online Learning Distractions

Some actions have a less positive effect on the neural networks in the brain. This was seen in 2020 when the COVID-19 pandemic struck. Schools were forced to close. Almost overnight the lives of millions of students were transformed as online classes replaced in-person learning. As classes moved onto computers, tablets, and phones, screen time doubled for many kids, according to Qustodio, a company that tracks device usage for children ages four to fifteen.

Lighting Up Brain Activity

A medical tool called magnetic resonance imaging (MRI) utilizes magnets, radio waves, and computers to capture detailed three-dimensional images of the brain and other parts of the body. Researchers who study the effects of social media use MRIs to map areas of the brain that are used when a person is performing various tasks, from studying to playing video games. These images can reveal parts of the brain most affected by tasks, thoughts, and emotions. The machine can also detect areas of the brain that are shrinking, growing, or changing over time due to excessive use of digital media.

MRI scans record heighted activity in a neural system within the brain known as the reward circuit. This network is active, for example, when subjects receive many likes on their social media posts. The reward circuitry links together brain structures that regulate the ability to feel pleasure. This is the same pathway activated when a person eats chocolate or wins money while gambling. While it might not be surprising that people experience pleasure when someone likes their photo, MRI helps scientists understand changes in the brains of those who cannot seem to put down their cell phones or game controllers.

The transition to virtual learning posed problems for those who found it difficult to pay attention when class was held on the Zoom video communications app. Some students suffered from what is known as Zoom burnout. This is the effect of staring at a computer screen for hours, which can result in exhaustion, stress, and even depression. The problem is due to the technology. Psychologist Brenda Wiederhold explains, "Our brains are used to picking up body language and other cues, not to mention increases of dopamine, that are experienced during face-to-face communication. On a video call, something is off, and our subconscious brain is reacting to that. Communication isn't in real time, even though we may think it is."[31] Fatigue is caused by the millisecond lag between the movement of a speaker's mouth and the words that are heard through headphones or speakers. The brain tires as it works to overcome this lack of synchronicity.

The Zoom classroom affects the brain in another way. Most videoconferences only frame a person's face, and this can be a problem on a large monitor. Viewers might subconsciously find it intimidating when the large face of a teacher or student appears before them. As Wiederhold explains, "When you have that large face in front of you or several large faces, it can ignite that fight-or-flight response . . . [and] your heart rate increase."[32]

The Emotional Quotient

While neural networks in student brains struggle to adapt to online learning, some argue that those who engage in excessive online video gaming seem to be causing their brains to shrink. This was put forth by researchers studying the grey matter of gamers. Grey matter is a substance that makes up the outer layer of the brain. Researchers focused on the area of the brain that sits above the eye sockets (the orbitofrontal cortex, or OFC). This region of the brain is used for impulse control and decision-making. The study compared the brains of people who had a history of excessive internet gaming with those who did not play video games. The gamers had less grey matter in the OFC region. Young people normally do not lose grey matter in this region; the loss is more common in older people who suffer from what is called age-related cognitive decline.

The study labeled this condition in young people internet gaming disorder. Those who suffer from this malady lack the ability to control their gaming addiction. They continue to excessively play video games despite the negative consequences of their behavior. And like those with age-related decline, their thinking seems to slow, and they have difficulty reading, retaining information, and paying attention.

Gaming and excessive digital distraction can also affect regions of the brain that control basic emotions. This ability, referred to as emotional intelligence, allows people to recognize and manage happiness, sadness, anger, excitement, and fear. Emotional intelligence also plays an important role in boosting creativity, the skill to form original thoughts and ideas in areas such as science, music, art, and literature.

Researchers measure emotional intelligence with a test called the Trait Emotional Intelligence Questionnaire. Test takers receive a score called an emotional quotient, or EQ. People with a high EQ are keenly aware of their own feelings and can recognize and understand emotions in others. They tend not to make impulsive decisions or react in anger when faced with a challenging situation. Business coach Brian Tait explains, "A high EQ makes you remain collected at the worst of times and helps you make decisions while understanding the emotions of the person you are dealing with, positively."[33]

According to researchers, people with a high EQ tend to be more successful in life. But EQ scores, like IQ scores, seem to be falling. In 2021 a study published in the *Journal of Personality* showed that college students in Australia, Canada, the United Kingdom, and the United States were becoming less emotionally intelligent. Researchers looked at seventy different studies with nearly seventeen thousand test subjects conducted during 2001 to 2019. They found that at least two facets of emotional intelligence were declining: well-being and self-control. The declines were stronger among males and those with greater access to technology. People who replaced face-to-face encounters with glowing blue screens were shown to be dulling the regions of their brain that allowed them to judge emotions in others and themselves.

While video games might lower a player's EQ, a 2020 study by Oxford University in the United Kingdom suggested that there are benefits connected with gaming. The study looked at players of two popular games, *Plants vs Zombies: Battle for Neighborville* and *Animal Crossing: New Horizons*. The study showed that players of these games were happier and had a more positive outlook. Other research has shown that some video games can improve memory, problem solving abilities, and concentration.

The Shopping Brain

Around 200 million people play video games worldwide, but gaming is not as popular as online shopping. In 2021 over 2.1

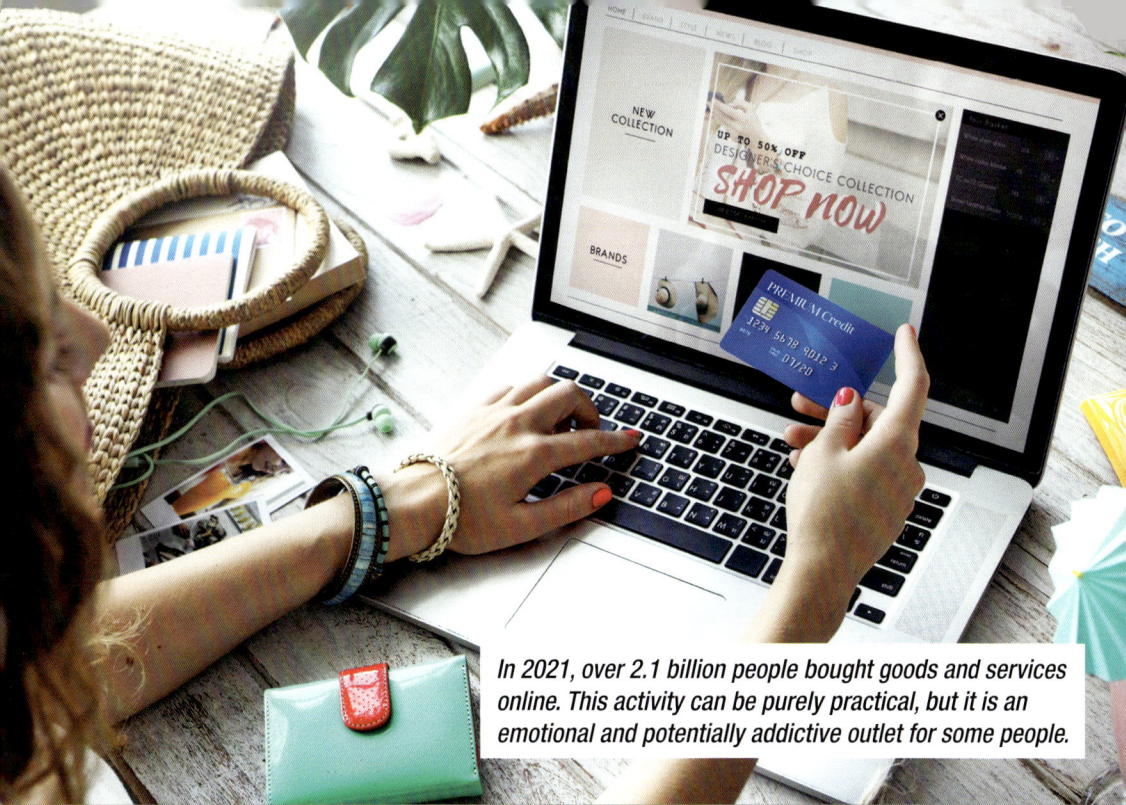

In 2021, over 2.1 billion people bought goods and services online. This activity can be purely practical, but it is an emotional and potentially addictive outlet for some people.

billion people bought goods and services online. This prompted scientists in the United Kingdom to examine the role that emotional intelligence plays in shopping. While many people consider purchasing goods online a necessary chore, British researchers found that it can also be an emotional task for some. Most shopping platforms use the same types of buzzes, flashes, pop-ups, and notifications seen on social media and online gaming sites. And the joy of purchasing a desired product can provide the same kind of dopamine rush as Instagram or TikTok. But shopping online can also be a frustrating experience. And this frustration can cause changes in the brain that make users feel disgusted, depressed, and even nauseated.

While online shopping is a relatively recent phenomenon, the experience can trigger regions of the brain that evolved around one hundred thousand years ago. Researchers at the University of London monitored the brain responses of test subjects using an electroencephalograph (EEG). An EEG uses electrodes placed on the scalp to detect electrical waves in the brain that

The Brain on Video Games

Studies have shown that excessive playing of violent video games can have negative effects on users, who might experience mood swings, insomnia, and trouble paying attention. These effects can be traced to areas of the brain that evolved to fight or flee when confronted with danger.

Many video games require users to strategize, survive attacks, accumulate weapons, fight, and kill. This intense visual and aural stimulation can trigger the brain to release a hormone called adrenaline from the adrenal glands above the kidneys. Adrenaline increases heart rate and directs blood to the limbs and heart. The brain becomes intensely aroused as it instructs the body to get ready to fight or escape. All this occurs while the player is at rest, moving little more than fingers and thumbs. Explaining why this is problematic, psychologist Victoria L. Dunckley says:

> When the fight-or-flight state occurs too often, or too intensely, the brain and body have trouble regulating themselves back to a calm state, leading to a state of chronic stress.... A hyperaroused and mentally depleted [gamer] will have trouble paying attention, managing emotions, suppressing impulses, following directions, tolerating frustration, accessing creativity and compassion, and executing tasks.

Victoria L. Dunckley, "This Is Your Child's Brain on Video Games," *Mental Wealth* (blog), *Psychology Today*, September 25, 2016. www.psychologytoday.com.

rise and fall as different neurons communicate with one another. Scientists also employed an electrocardiograph, a machine to monitor the heart activity of test subjects. Researchers presented test subjects with online shopping scenarios that were meant to be very frustrating. These included having a wedding dress delivered a day late, after the wedding. In a second scenario users spent an hour online waiting to purchase concert tickets only to have the website crash when they were next in line. Another situation involved having a highly desired product returned to the sender because the shopper's address was incorrect.

The EEG imaging showed that these unpleasant online shopping experiences stimulated activity in the part of the brain known as the anterior insula. This region is active when people feel disgust after exposure to offensive smells, tastes, or images. Being disgusted is basic to survival; humans evolved the emotion so they would avoid rotting food, dead and decaying organisms, harmful insects like cockroaches, and bodily waste products.

The test revealed that people are highly reactive to bad online experiences. Neuroscientist Jack Lewis, who helped conduct the experiment, explains the results. "Not only do consumers vividly recall their own highly frustrating online retail experiences," he says, "but as these memories flood back they are accompanied by changes in the brain and heart data that indicate an urge to flee. This . . . [indicates] that frustrations in the context of online retail are powerfully repellant."[34]

> "Consumers vividly recall their own highly frustrating online retail experiences, but as these memories flood back they are accompanied by changes in the brain and heart data that indicate an urge to flee."[34]
>
> —Jack Lewis, neuroscientist

Evolution of the Mind

Scientific studies about the effects of the internet on the brain have shown that the digital world might be rearranging people's grey matter. But research also offers hope; brain plasticity works both ways. When a person replaces addictive scrolling or excessive gaming with making art or reading books, their brain functions return to a more natural state.

It is doubtful that billions of people are going to put down their smartphones in favor of painting or writing novels. But the brain is the most intricate computer in the world. It will continue to adapt and evolve as it has over thousands of years, absorbing the flood of digital information and processing it. And people will need to better understand how the online world can alter their brains.

CHAPTER THREE

The Myth and Reality of Multitasking

Some people are heavy multitaskers. They spend their days texting, shopping online, posting selfies to social media, watching TV, and playing video games, sometimes all at once. In the car they might be drinking coffee, tweaking the entertainment system, and making phone calls while maneuvering their vehicle through traffic. (They are probably breaking the law if they are holding the phone while driving; it is illegal in most states.) When multitaskers get to work or school, they might continue their activities on smartphones, laptops, tablets, and desktop computers.

Many heavy multitaskers are proud of their abilities. When filling out résumés or sitting through job interviews, they emphasize that they are good at multitasking. And many employers expect their workers to juggle several tasks at once. But numerous studies have shown that most people are not good at multitasking. Multitaskers are less productive and more prone to error, and they tire faster than those who focus on one task at a time. And multitasking can make life more difficult. Writer Hayley Phelan says that multitasking is essential to her job, but "if I keep looking at my phone or my inbox or various websites, working feels a lot more tortuous. When I'm focused and making progress, work is actually pleasurable."[35]

The Cost of Switching

Basic brain functions make true multitasking nearly impossible for most people. When the brain is focused on a single task, portions of both frontal lobes are active. When a second task is added, the brain suffers from what neuroscientists call interference; the tasks compete for finite thinking resources in the same areas of the brain. Interference acts as a bottleneck that clogs the transfer of information between portions of the brain. When a third task is added, one will effectively be forgotten; the brain carries on by ignoring it. Neuroscientist Earl Miller affirms, "Your brain can only produce one or two thoughts [at once]. . . . We're very, very single-minded. [We have] very limited cognitive capacity."[36]

Miller says average teenagers believe they can simultaneously follow six forms of media. But like almost all multitaskers, they are instead switching back and forth between media sources. Their brains only focus on one at a time. As Miller explains, "They don't notice the switching because their brain sort of papers it over to give a seamless experience of consciousness, but what they're actually doing is switching and reconfiguring their brain moment-to-moment, task-to-task"[37] According to Miller, all that switching comes with a cost. Thought processes become scattered and slow.

> "Your brain can only produce one or two thoughts [at once]. . . . We're very, very single-minded. [We have] very limited cognitive capacity."[36]
>
> —Earl Miller, neuroscientist

Scientists have a term for this drop in mental performance; the switch-cost effect. It defines the price paid in accuracy and efficiency when switching attention between several forms of media. The switch-cost effect comes into play when a student is doing homework but stops to check the phone for an Instagram update. While this action only takes a few seconds, research shows it can take up to twenty minutes for the student to effectively refocus on homework after an interruption.

The switch-cost effect was first demonstrated in 2013 by researchers at Carnegie Mellon University's Human-Computer Interaction Lab when 136 students were given a standard test. Some had their phones switched off while other received short text messages during the test period. Those who got texts performed 20 percent worse on the test than those who did not. This increase in errors is called the screw-up effect. Miller says switching between tasks causes mistakes that would not have occurred otherwise. "Your brain is error-prone," he explains. "When you switch from task to task, your brain has to backtrack a little bit and pick up and figure out where it left off [and glitches start to occur]. . . . Instead of spending critical time really doing deep thinking, your thinking is more superficial, because you're spending a lot of time correcting errors and backtracking."[38]

Bad Taskers and Supertaskers

Despite the research, many believe they are expert multitaskers. This type of overconfidence is known as cognitive bias. It defines the tendency of individuals to overrate their skills in any situation. And those who have cognitive bias are too overconfident to realize when they are making obvious mistakes.

Individuals with cognitive bias can be found in almost every social and intellectual environment. They overrate their skills as students, teachers, professionals, and entertainers. And a 2018 study reported in the journal *Proceedings of the National Academy of Sciences* showed that cognitive bias is extremely common among heavy multitaskers. Subjects who claimed to be very good at multitasking were asked to perform several tasks at once, such as memorizing word combinations while operating a car-driving simulator. Those with cognitive bias did much worse on tests than those who did not overrate their abilities.

A team of psychologists at the University of Utah found a surprising exception to the cognitive bias rule. A small percentage of people who highly rate their own skills are observably better at multitasking than almost everyone else. Researchers in Utah discovered that a little over 2 percent of the population can be classified as supertaskers. The performance of supertaskers improves when they are completing multiple tasks at once. The brains of supertaskers operate differently; when they are multitasking, there is less activity in the frontal lobes, rather than more.

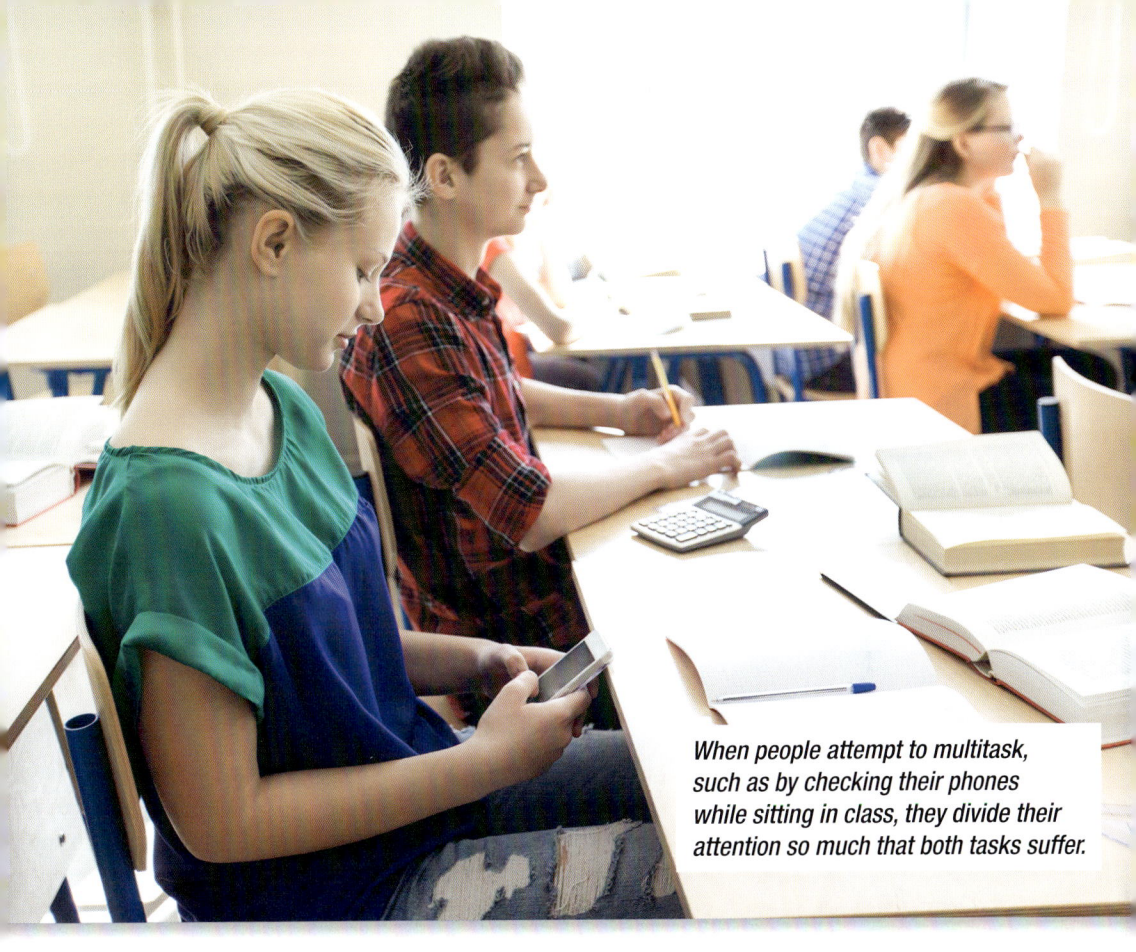

When people attempt to multitask, such as by checking their phones while sitting in class, they divide their attention so much that both tasks suffer.

This means the brains of supertaskers become less active with additional tasks. While researchers do not fully understand how this works, they believe that this lower level of activity allows the brains of supertaskers to work more efficiently. As psychology professor and lead author of the study David Strayer says, "Their brains are doing something we can't do."[39]

One of the supertaskers in Strayer's study is known as Cassie. She was able to operate a driving simulator, do math problems, and listen to commands being given to her through a cell phone. While most people failed the test after a few minutes, Cassie seemed to be getting more efficient. Strayer explained, "It's a really, really hard test. Some people come out woozy—'I have a headache'. . . that sort of thing. But she solved everything. . . . She made zero mistakes. And she did even better when she was driving."[40]

Scientists speculate that supertaskers like Cassie are rare because there are few evolutionary benefits related to performing more than one mental task at a time. As technology becomes even more embedded in everyone's daily lives, more people might evolve into supertaskers. But for now, supertaskers are an exception.

Phishing for Multitaskers

People can fool themselves into thinking they are good at multitasking, but online fraudsters know better. These criminals, who conduct phishing attacks and phone scams, understand that distracted multitaskers make easy targets. Scammers produce millions of emails, SMS texts, and robocalls every day to lure the digitally distracted into giving away passwords, personal information, and money.

Internet crime increased nearly 70 percent in 2020, according to the Federal Bureau of Investigation. And the tactics of phishers became more sophisticated. Scammers fool the public by using names and logos of banks, government tax bureaus, and law enforcement agencies. They might pretend to be a lawyer, doctor, or family member in need of urgent financial help. And mobile devices are the main scammer target. When compared to large computer monitors, smartphone screens are small. Tiny message boxes make it difficult for some to see the names, links, and web addresses sent by fraudsters. And people are so busy multitasking that they might click on a harmful link by accident. A 2018 study from Michigan State University showed that people switch apps over one hundred times a day. This means they are not paying attention to details. Professor of decision sciences Cleotilde Gonzalez says, "If you are on an iPhone, looking at a Facebook message or quickly trying to figure out what an SMS is telling you, there is a higher chance that you are going to fall into the trap of a phishing attempt."[41]

> "If you are [multitasking], there is a higher chance that you are going to fall into the trap of a phishing attempt."[41]
>
> —Cleotilde Gonzalez, professor of decision sciences

Multitasking and Homework

Multitasking has been shown to have negative consequences on productivity, health, and behavior. But a 2019 study by Ohio State University discovered that multitasking can also help adolescents feel better about the main task they are trying to accomplish. Young people ages eleven to seventeen were given a task they did not want to do—their homework. Researchers found that those who texted with friends while doing homework felt better about the chore while multitasking. However, the pleasant feelings decreased after a while as more mental energy was needed to multitask.

The study also showed that those who were performing rewarding tasks, such as drawing or playing music, felt less desire to multitask. Professor of communications Zheng Wang, who coauthored the study, explains the findings: "It suggests that adolescents may be less likely to multitask if they already find their tasks rewarding. Efforts by teachers to make lectures more interactive and efforts by parents to engage children in activities that offer opportunities to play, explore and learn all should help reduce multitasking."

Zheng Wang et al., "Multitasking and Dual Motivational Systems: A Dynamic Longitudinal Study," *Human Communication Research*, October 2019. https://academic.oup.com.

When it comes to online fraud, cognitive bias once again comes into play. Most people think they are too sophisticated to get scammed. And there is a stereotype that only gullible older people are tricked by cybercriminals. The reality is that older people spend less time with digital devices and are more distrustful of messages from people they do not know. That is why phishers most often target young people, who generally spend more time online. According to psychologist Gareth Norris, "Younger people use technology all the time, they're on the phones all the time. And actually, they give information out quite freely, and they're not too worried about it."[42]

Deadly Multitasking

Multitasking can turn from dangerous to deadly when the smartphones are used by people driving vehicles. When drivers send or read texts, they take their eyes off the road for at least five seconds. A car traveling at 60 miles an hour (96.6 kph) covers around a tenth of a mile (160 m) during that short period of time. This prompted the National Highway Traffic Safety Administration (NHTSA) to say that those who drive while texting have the same level of reaction impairment as a drunk driver who consumed four beers within an hour. Texting drivers are twenty times more likely to get into an accident than those who aren't texting.

Texting while driving is illegal in all fifty states, but the NHTSA says around 660,000 people in the United States are using a cell phone while driving at any given moment. While not all are texting, 46 percent of sixteen- and seventeen-year-olds admit to text messaging while driving. And 10 percent of adults and 20 percent of teens admit to having multiple text conversations while operating a motor vehicle. In most states any driver under age eighteen is prohibited from using a cell phone for any purpose while operating a car.

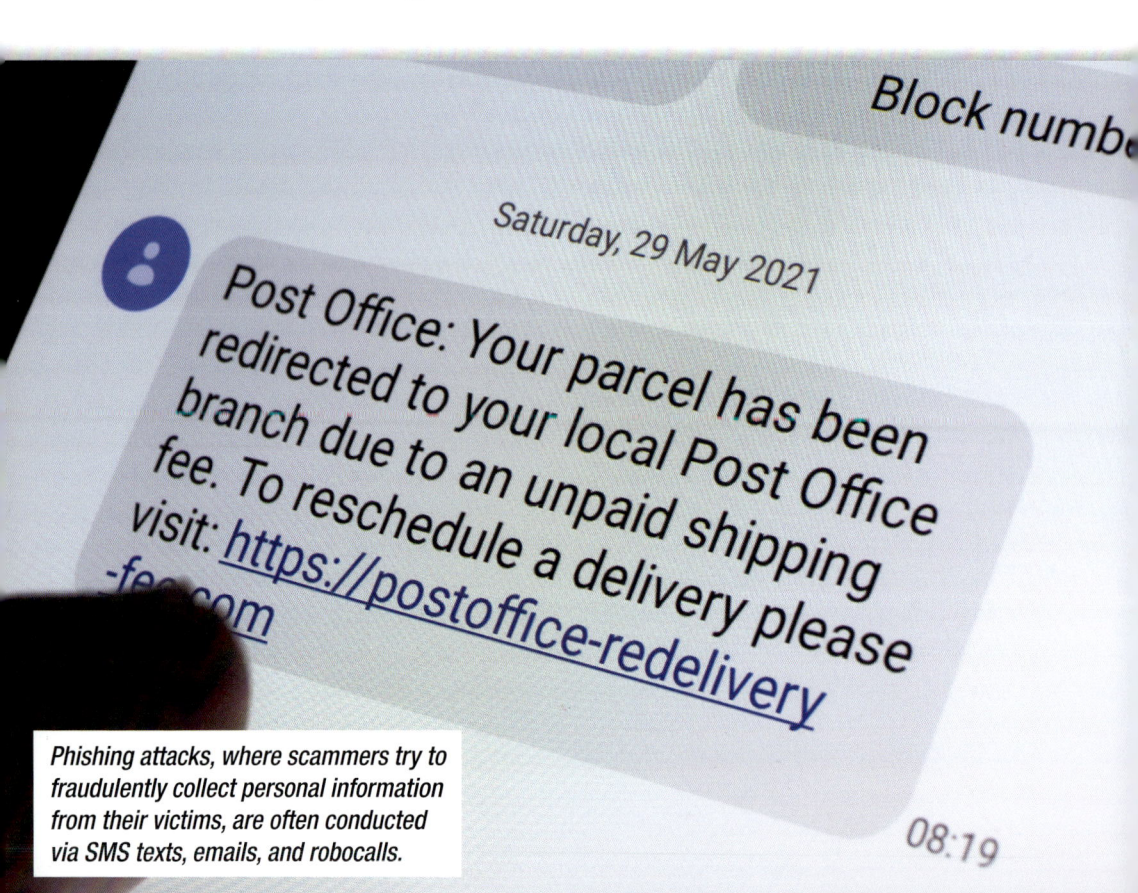

Phishing attacks, where scammers try to fraudulently collect personal information from their victims, are often conducted via SMS texts, emails, and robocalls.

Alexandra Mansonet understands the dangers of texting while driving only too well. Mansonet was piloting her Mercedes-Benz down a winding two-lane road in New Jersey several miles from her home when she received a text. Her sister-in-law wanted to know what kind of food she wanted for dinner, Cuban, Mexican, or American. Mansonet was in the middle of replying to the text when she plowed into a Toyota that was stopped at stop sign. The Toyota was pushed into a pedestrian, thirty-nine-year-old Yu-wen Wang, who died five days later. When police arrived at the scene of the accident, Mansonet told them, "I looked up and the car was right in front of me."[43] She turned her phone over to police, who read an unsent text with the letters "m" and "e" still in the reply box. In 2019 Mansonet was charged with violating a New Jersey law that equates texting while driving with drunk driving. In 2020 she was convicted of vehicular homicide and received a five-year prison sentence.

The dangers of cell phone use while driving are not limited to texting. Simply talking on the phone while driving leads to longer braking times, inattention to road signals, and dangerous behavior like tailgating. These problems occur even when the driver is not holding the phone and his or her eyes are on the road ahead.

Deadly car accidents are an extreme example of the harm that can result from multitasking. Other problems, while less disastrous, can affect the long-term health of multitaskers. A 2019 study published in the journal *Brain Imaging and Behavior* showed that performing multiple tasks at once can be unhealthy. Researchers using MRIs saw that multitasking can cause a chemical imbalance in the brain that increases the appetite. As a result, young multitaskers who rapidly switch between forms of digital media are more susceptible to becoming overweight or obese. Multitasking also causes memory problems, increases stress, and even harms romantic relationships.

Experts say those who wish to avoid the pitfalls of multitasking can learn to work more efficiently. Data scientist Chan Priya recommends listing tasks in order of importance: "Once you

Negative Emotions and Multitasking

Some people find it relaxing to multitask with several forms of media. But a 2020 study by the University of Houston found that multitasking in the workplace can lead to negative emotions like fear and sadness. Researchers created an algorithm to analyze the emotions expressed on the faces of tech workers as they concentrated on writing an essay. One group of test subjects answered a batch of emails before they began writing, while a second group was required to answer emails that continually interrupted their main task. While the expressions of subjects in the first group remained neutral, those who were interrupted seemed to suffer. Professor of computer science Ioannis Pavlidis, who authored the study, explains, "Individuals who engaged in multitasking appeared significantly sadder than those who did not. Interestingly, sadness tended to mix with a touch of fear. . . . Multitasking imposes an onerous mental load and is associated with elevated stress, which appears to trigger the displayed sadness." Pavlidis says that negative emotions displayed in the workplace can be contagious; they tend to spread throughout the entire office, creating an undesirable environment for everyone.

Quoted in Sara Tubbs, "Multitasking in the Workplace Can Lead to Negative Emotions," University of Houston, May 11, 2020. https://uh.edu.

prioritize the things, you have a clear idea of what needs to be done and when. . . . You can decide what order to do things by thinking about which tasks are urgent and how important each task is."[44] Priya recommends trying to ignore tasks that are not on the list, such as updating an Instagram account or texting a friend about dinner.

Computers and Humans

The problems caused by multitasking are not going away. Many people are required to multitask just to get through the day. Research by the Department of Informatics at the University of California, Irvine, discovered that a typical office worker is distracted every three minutes during the workday. Best-selling author Johann Hari reports on the study:

The average office worker now spends 40 percent of their work time wrongly believing they are "multitasking"—which means they are incurring all these costs for their attention and focus. In fact, uninterrupted time is becoming rare. . . . Most of us working in offices never get a whole hour uninterrupted in a normal day. . . . This is happening at every level of businesses—the average [chief executive officer] of a Fortune 500 company, for example, gets just twenty-eight uninterrupted minutes a day.[45]

Hari points out that the term *multitasking*, while widely used, is not an accurate term for human behavior. The word first appeared in print in 1965 to describe what was then an advanced IBM computer that could simultaneously run several programs. Ironically, the computer was mimicking the human brain; it was switching back and forth between tasks, but at a much faster rate

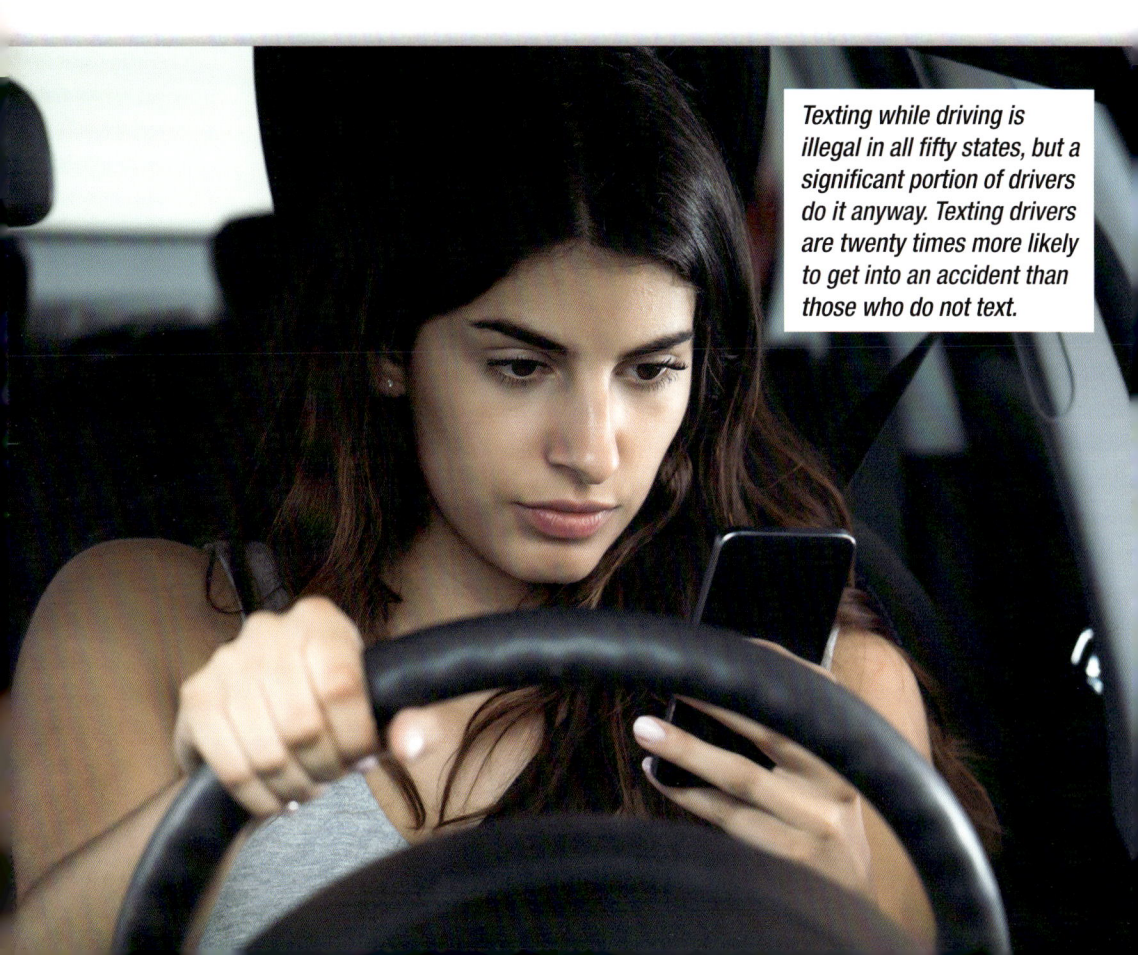

Texting while driving is illegal in all fifty states, but a significant portion of drivers do it anyway. Texting drivers are twenty times more likely to get into an accident than those who do not text.

> "The ninety-eight per cent of us, we deceive ourselves. And we tend to overrate our ability to multitask."[46]
>
> —David Strayer, psychology professor

than a brain. This process, called context switching, is still used in modern computers that perform multiple tasks so rapidly that they seem to be doing everything at once.

Computers have advanced to the point that they are carried around in people's pocket or purse in the form of smartphones. But the brain has not changed. Most people can best get things done by doing what researchers call single-tasking or monotasking—doing just one thing at a time. As Strayer states, "The ninety-eight per cent of us, we deceive ourselves. And we tend to overrate our ability to multitask."[46]

The research is clear, but it is doubtful that people will radically change their behavior as the pop-ups, direct messages, TV shows, music streaming, and social media continue to beckon. But as British author Jeremy Clarkson says, the accurate term for multitasking should be *mistake-tasking*: "Multitasking is the ability to screw everything up simultaneously."[47]

CHAPTER FOUR

Time for a Digital Detox?

There is little doubt that digital devices, social media apps, and online shopping sites are specifically designed to grab people's attention. And digital overload is a defining problem of modern life. Anyone sitting in a classroom, office, restaurant, or almost any other public place can see numerous people with their noses buried in their smartphones. They are most likely being bombarded with messages and alerts that make it nearly impossible to focus on what is going on around them.

Many people feel that resistance is futile. Everything they do—including learning, working, socializing, and consuming entertainment—relies on an internet connection and a digital device. But all that digital diversion comes at a price. The Pew Research Center reports that around half of all teens feel as if they are addicted to their smartphones. The phone is the first thing they reach for in the morning and the last thing they look at before bed. And around one-third say they check their phones in the middle of the night. But the internet, which interrupts so much concentration, has numerous groups fighting to reduce society's digital attention deficit. Some, like the National Day of Unplugging, only ask that people turn off their phones one day a year, on the first Friday in March.

Going on a Digital Diet

Turning off a smartphone for a day might not seem like much, but Reviews.org reports that 53 percent of Americans have never gone twenty-four hours without looking at their phones. For many in this group, it is just not realistic to cut off all communications with their family, friends, or job. This motivates some go on a digital diet to reduce their phone use and make it more manageable.

Those who do succeed at reducing digital distraction report many positive effects. Kevin Roose discovered this in 2019, as he wrote in the *New York Times*: "I ditched my phone and unbroke my brain."[48] Roose is a technology reporter, and his job requires him to take deep dives into the digital world daily. But like many of the digitally distracted, he found it increasingly difficult to read a book, watch an entire movie, or concentrate on a conversation.

> "I ditched my phone and unbroke my brain."[48]
>
> —Kevin Roose, tech journalist

Roose blamed his smartphone for his attention deficit. This led him to take several steps that can be beneficial to anyone wishing to cut back on their smartphone habit. The first thing Roose did was to turn on the Screen Time feature in his iPhone settings so he could analyze exactly how much time he spent on his phone. He was horrified to learn that he picked up his phone 101 times in a single day and spent 5 hours and 37 minutes using it for various purposes. The results prompted Roose to set up what he called mental speed bumps that would force him to think for a moment before he picked up the phone. Some simply put a rubber band around their device. This reminds them to pause for a few moments before engaging with their phone. Roose had a different approach; he changed his lock screen to feature a meme with three questions he would ask himself before using the phone: "What for? Why Now? What Else?"[49]

After changing his settings, Roose became keenly aware that he was uncomfortable during quiet moments. This led him to increase his awareness of his surroundings. When he walked to work, he looked up at the buildings and made note of interesting architectural details. He watched people on the

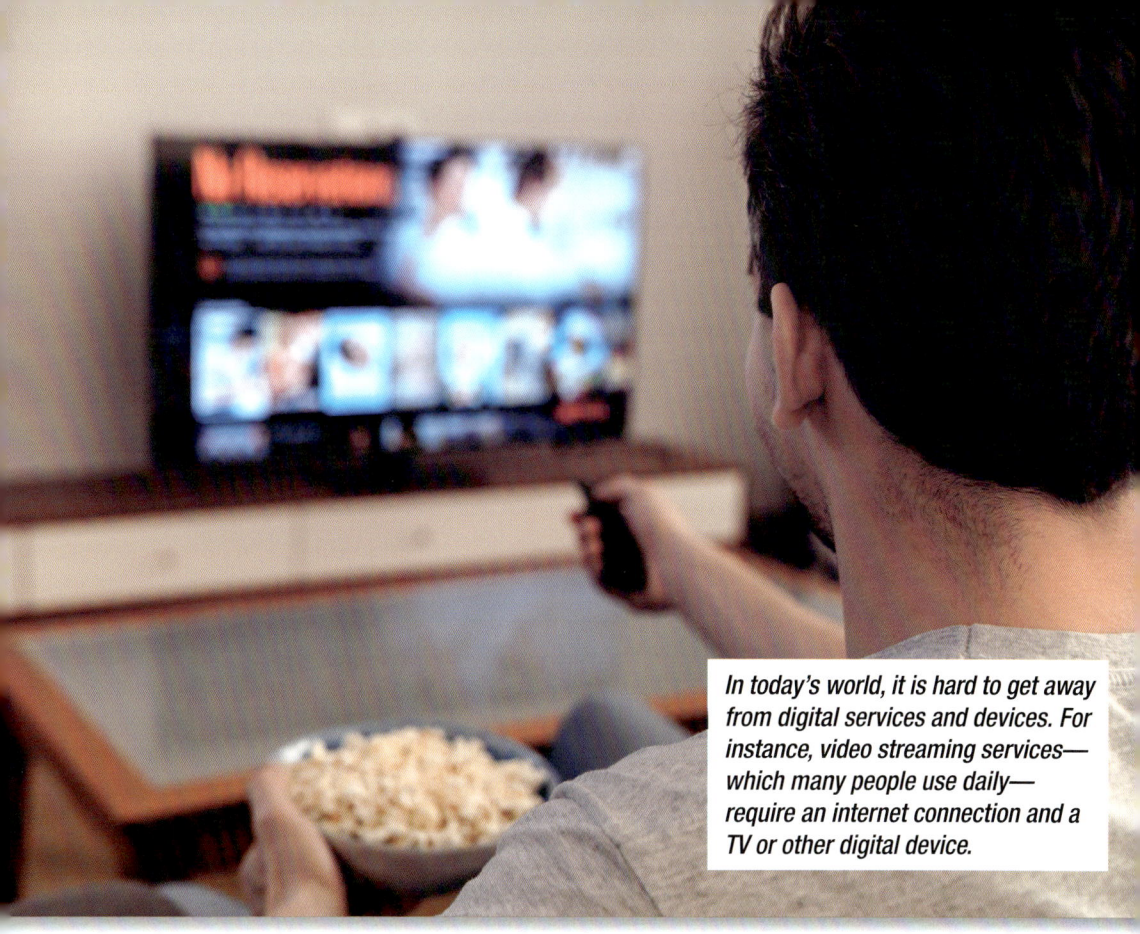

In today's world, it is hard to get away from digital services and devices. For instance, video streaming services—which many people use daily—require an internet connection and a TV or other digital device.

subway, just enjoying how people dressed and interacted. But by paying attention to the world around him, he noticed something disturbing—most people in public are staring at their phones like zombies.

Ditch Apps, Find a Hobby

Experts say going on a smartphone diet involves the difficult step of deleting all the apps that do not contribute to healthy habits. This led Roose to ditch Twitter, Facebook, YouTube, news apps, and games. He kept the basic apps that are used for navigation, appointments, and email. Back in his settings, he turned off notifications for everything except phone calls from a short list of people, including his boss, family, and close friends.

While Roose kept his iPhone, some go on a digital diet by trading their smartphone for what might be called a dumbphone.

The National Day of Unplugging

The National Day of Unplugging holds an annual event during which people turn off all their digital devices for twenty-four hours. The unplugging runs from sundown on the first Friday in March to sundown the next day. In 2021 the organization reported that people in thirty-seven countries participated in the event by unplugging for at least twenty-four hours.

Participants in the National Day of Unplugging are encouraged to engage in family activities such as painting rocks with positive messages, hosting a household comedy night, playing board games, or holding a scavenger hunt. Some use the event to raise money for charities by signing up sponsors for an Unplug-A-Thon. During the National Day of Unplugging, individuals organize nature walks, yoga sessions, rock-climbing expeditions, and bike tours. As author David Sax explains on the National Day of Unplugging website, "Remember that unplugging isn't some test to endure for a day, like a fast. It is permission to indulge in a way of communicating, interacting, and relaxing with the tangible world that can be more rewarding, and enjoyable, than whatever you won't miss on your phone."

David Sax, "Unplug . . . Then What?," National Day of Unplugging, October 27, 2017. www.nationaldayofunplugging.com.

Makers of one such device, the Light Phone II, intend it to be used by those who are trying to wean themselves from their smartphones. The relatively inexpensive Light Phone II is small and sleek like an iPhone, but has extremely limited features that make it useless for downloading apps or surfing the internet. The phone has a simple music player and can be used to make phone calls, send texts, set an alarm, or provide directions.

The dumbphone has a paper-like screen like those found on e-readers. Unlike a smartphone, it does not emit blue light, which has been shown to disrupt sleep patterns when used late at night. Studies show that sleep can also be disrupted just by keeping a phone next to the bed. Some avoid this by storing their phones in a room far from the bedroom. Roose took the extraordinary step of buying a mini safe in which to stash his phone at a set time every night. He said this step helped him cut down on his phone usage while he was at home with his family.

Many who want to reduce their digital overload pick up new hobbies when they put down the phone. The healing power of art is well known. People who express themselves through music, art, writing, and other creative endeavors have better powers of concentration and are less likely to experience anxiety, depression, and insomnia. Engaging in physical activities like hiking, biking, and sports can also improve mental and physical health. Roose found that pottery was a perfect substitute for his smartphone: "It's manually challenging and demands concentration for hours on end. It gets your hands dirty, too, which is a good deterrent to fiddling with expensive electronics."[50]

Even after all the steps he took on his digital diet, Roose was still having trouble disconnecting. But his wife was much happier; he no longer ignored her in favor of texting and surfing for the latest celebrity news. The action of snubbing someone in favor of using a phone is known as "phubbing." Those who engage in excessive phubbing are less happy in their relationships and more prone to feel depressed and alienated.

After a month of digital detoxing, Roose found that he was using his iPhone for about an hour a day and picked it up only twenty times. He said he felt as if something had shifted in his brain. He recalls:

> A few weeks ago, the world on my phone seemed more compelling than the offline world—more colorful, faster-moving and with a bigger scope of rewards. . . . Now, the physical world excites me, too—the one that has room for boredom, idle hands and space for thinking. . . . I look people in the eye and listen when they talk. . . . And when I get sucked into my phone, I notice and self-correct.[51]

Taking Time Off

While Roose exhibited a great level of self-control, most young people lack the discipline necessary to go on a digital diet. Many will not even consider turning off their phones, even for a day. But on some occasions teens can be convinced to give up their phones as part of an experiment. In 2018 philosophy professor Ron Srigley offered students extra class credit if they would surrender their smartphones for nine days. After the experiment, they had to write about their digitally disconnected life.

Srigley teaches at Humber College in Toronto. He was motivated to conduct the test after most students in his class did poorly on their midterm exams. When Srigley asked students what went wrong, many agreed that they could not understand the words in the textbook. Srigley believed they would do better if they put down their phones.

Twelve of Srigley's thirty-six students participated in the experiment. He said that most initially felt lost, frustrated, and disoriented without their phones. Some were even frightened to go out in the world without their devices. But after a few days, most of them realized that their phones were limiting their real-life experiences and cutting them off from others. A student named Stewart explained his feelings: "Being forced to have [real relations with people] obviously made me a better person because each time it happened I learned how to deal with the situation better, other than sticking my face in a phone."[52]

> "[Having real relations with people] made me a better person because each time it happened I learned how to deal with the situation better, other than sticking my face in a phone."[52]
>
> —Stewart, college student

Many of those who stopped using their phones experienced relief. Eight of the students said they were happy to be freed from answering a constant flood of texts and social media posts. Some came to see the constant alerts, pop-ups, and vibrations as a form of harassment that they were glad to be rid of. Stewart said that without the constant digital irritations, he was able to focus better on his work: "I was able to give it 100% of my attention, not only was the final product better than it would have been, I was also able to complete it much quicker."[53]

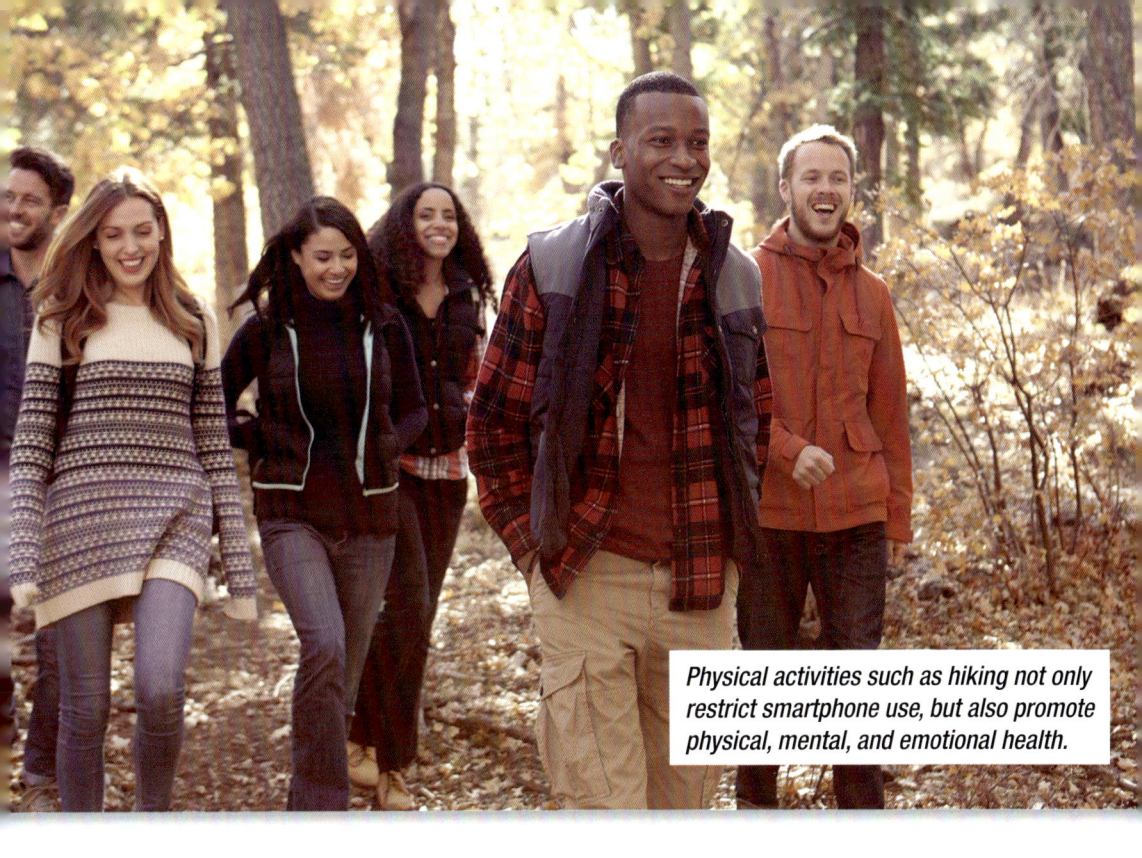

Physical activities such as hiking not only restrict smartphone use, but also promote physical, mental, and emotional health.

While tech companies sell their products as a way for everyone to stay connected, studies show that constant use of digital devices increases feelings of isolation and loneliness. Students who surrendered their phones felt more connected to one another. They looked each other in the eye when having a conversation, and there was no phubbing in awkward situations. However, a participant named Emily found out what it was like to be phubbed when she simply walked by strangers in the school hallway or street, which she says led "almost all of them to take out a phone right before I could gain eye contact with them."[54]

Reducing Digital Dependence

Srigley's experiment was informal and did not focus on steps students could take to reduce their digital dependence. However, scientists, researchers, and tech companies have studied the issue of social media and smartphone addiction and have developed a series of steps users can take to help them set limits on their screen time.

One of the first steps involves consciously thinking about scrolling rather than doing it thoughtlessly. This concept is based on a 2018 Australian study in which 86 percent of adults said they scrolled automatically. They mindlessly pulled out their phones while waiting in a checkout line, sitting in a restaurant, riding on an elevator, or even waiting for a red light when driving. To counteract this activity, experts recommend setting aside a specific time for scrolling and sticking to the schedule. If users know that they will be scrolling between 6:00 and 7:00 p.m. every day, for example, they will be more aware, or mindful, of the activity. Professor of business management Arthur C. Brooks claims that establishing a scrolling schedule is a good idea. He explains, "The best way to counteract mindless scrolling is with mindful scrolling. Set times each day or week to look at your smartphone and really focus on it. Don't do anything else; be all about the phone for those minutes, as if it were your job. . . . Besides making addiction easier to beat . . . such a practice might also show you how little you actually enjoy staring at your phone."[55]

> "The best way to counteract mindless scrolling is with mindful scrolling. Set times each day or week to look at your smartphone and really focus on it."[55]
>
> —Arthur C. Brooks, professor of business management

Users can be more mindful of their behavior if they establish phone-free periods each day. The best time to do this is when engaged in other activities. Turning off the phone during dinner, while watching a film, or when socializing with friends and family allows users to focus on the moment instead of being sidetracked by the latest mindless comment on Instagram or TikTok.

Another way to reduce digital disruption is to disable notifications. These alerts, which trigger the release of dopamine in the brain, are addictive. Checking even a single notification can lead to an extended period of scrolling. According to Brooks, "Smartphones game our dopamine, most crucially through

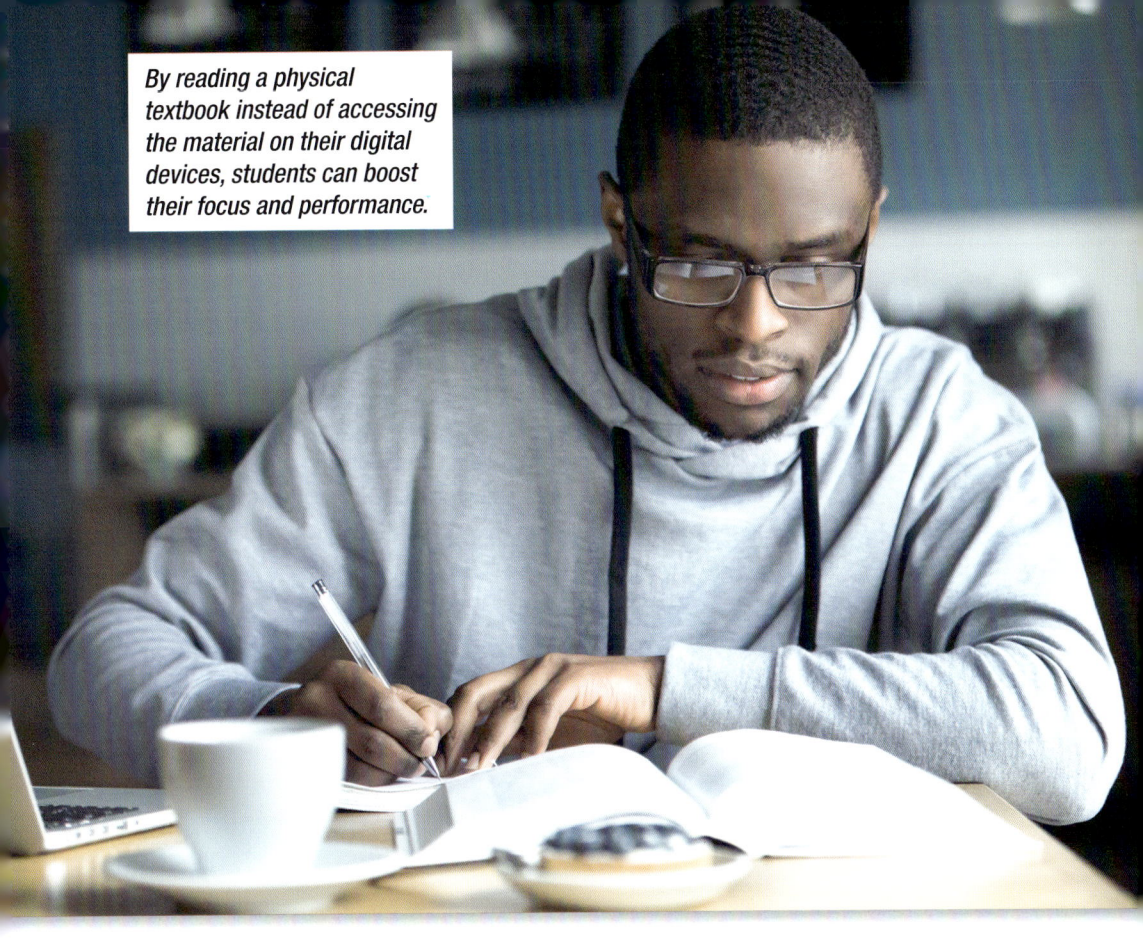

By reading a physical textbook instead of accessing the material on their digital devices, students can boost their focus and performance.

the sounds and banners indicating that someone messaged or mentioned you and you must look right now to satisfy your curiosity."[56]

Apps That Fight Apps

Smartphones all come with settings that can help users stick to their digital diets. The iPhone Screen Time setting allows users to set a schedule for time away from the screen. Users can set daily time limits for apps and categories they want to manage. The app provides a weekly report that reveals exactly how much time is spent on the phone. The app, for example, includes a passcode that parents can use to control the amount of time a child spends on the device. Adults who are trying to cut back on digital distractions can also give that passcode to their spouses or friends, who can use it to control the owner's phone time.

Hold Calls with This App

App designer Maths Mathisen came up with a fun way to break his phone addiction. When Mathisen was a college student in Norway in 2020, he was constantly distracted from his studies by the notifications emanating from his phone. He decided to have a contest with his friends to see how long they could go without checking their phones. The person who lost would have to buy coffee for everyone in the group. This game prompted Mathisen to invent an app called Hold that makes turning off the phone a game. Users of the free app can sign up their friends and family to engage in a friendly competition to see who can go the longest without checking a phone. The app also works on desktop computers so users can follow the progress of others without picking up the phone. Mathisen explained why he was motivated to create Hold: "You spent 76 days on your phone per year. Think about if you can turn that into more productive work. You probably don't have a friend that you spent 76 days a year with. . . . [Our willpower] needs to be better than ever. That's hard if you don't have a way to control it."

Quoted in Penny Zenker, "The Productivity Toll You Need to Get a Hold of with Maths Mathisen," The Focusologist, November 6, 2020. https://pennyzenker360.com.

In addition to phone settings, there are apps that help users unplug. AppDetox lets users schedule phone downtime for physical activities and allows them to limit the number of launches for specific apps. When users violate their own rules, AppDetox reminds them to take a break and stop heavy phone usage. The app Flipd takes a more aggressive approach to help users stay focused. Flipd comes with a Full Lock setting that hides social media apps and games. The app cannot be unlocked during the scheduled period even if the phone is restarted.

Some digital detox apps use rewards to help people curtail their phone habit. Users of Forest set an amount of time they want to spend away from their device. The app plants a virtual tree that grows and thrives during that time. The tree dies if the user checks the phone before the allotted time period. The Forest app lets users see a catalog of their wins and losses at a glance. Those who are successful are awarded virtual coins. These coins can be spent to grow real forests. The Forest app partners with the organization Trees for the Future, which had planted over 2 million trees as of early 2022, paid for with redeemed coins.

Start a Healthy Relationship

Millions who use apps for digital detoxing report positive results. The apps help users become more mindful of how much time they spend on their devices. This alone has been shown to help people reduce their digital use. And the apps are needed now more than ever. Between school, work, and their personal lives, countless people spend the bulk of their waking hours online. And the average US smartphone user receives forty-six push notifications a day, according to the mobile marketing company CleverTap. If each notification causes only four minutes of disruption, this adds up to more than three hours of digital distraction each day, or twenty-one hours per week.

Maths Mathisen, inventor of the app Hold, which helps people break their phone addiction, believes it is important for people to take back control of their lives. "I want us to have a healthy relationship with our smartphones, tablets and laptops, using them only when necessary and to add value whenever they are used," he says. "I would like to work towards a world where the emphasis is on human interactions, as opposed to virtual ones, where people spend less time with their phone and more quality time with their loved ones."[57] Breaking any bad habit requires work. But the rewards of putting down the phone and seeing the world through fresh eyes can make the effort worthwhile.

> "I would like to work towards a world where the emphasis is on human interactions, as opposed to virtual ones, where people spend less time with their phone and more quality time with their loved ones."[57]
>
> —Maths Mathisen, app developer

SOURCE NOTES

Introduction: Smartphones and Ancient Brains

1. Quoted in OrthoInfo, "Distracted Walking," 2021. https://orthoinfo.aaos.org.
2. Derek Thompson, "Social Media Is Attention Alcohol," *The Atlantic*, September 17, 2021. www.theatlantic.com.
3. Quoted in Kenneth Miller, "How Our Ancient Brains Are Coping in the Age of Digital Distraction," *Discover*, April 20, 2020. www.discovermagazine.com.
4. Quoted in Mary Gillis, "Average Person Touches Their Smartphone 2,617 Times per Day, High Number Linked to 'Brain Drain,'" WISHTV, June 28, 2021. www.wishtv.com.
5. Quoted in Ira Flatow, "Decoding 'the Most Complex Object in the Universe,'" NPR, June 14, 2013. www.npr.org.
6. Quoted in Miller, "How Our Ancient Brains Are Coping in the Age of Digital Distraction."

Chapter One: Digitally Connected 24/7

7. Quoted in Paul Lewis, "'Our Minds Can Be Hijacked': The Tech Insiders Who Fear Smartphone Dystopia," *The Guardian* (Manchester, UK), October 6, 2017. www.theguardian.com.
8. Quoted in Scraps from the Loft, "*The Social Dilemma* (2020)—Transcript," October 3, 2020. https://scrapsfromtheloft.com.
9. Quoted in Janna Anderson and Lee Rainie, "The Negatives of Digital Life," Pew Research Center, July 3, 2018. www.pewresearch.org.
10. Quoted in Anderson and Rainie, "The Negatives of Digital Life."
11. Quoted in Hanna Schwär, "How Instagram and Facebook Are Intentionally Designed to Mimic Addictive Painkillers," Business Insider, August 11, 2021. www.businessinsider.com.
12. Quoted in Schwär, "How Instagram and Facebook Are Intentionally Designed to Mimic Addictive Painkillers."
13. Quoted in Scraps from the Loft, "*The Social Dilemma* (2020)—Transcript."
14. Quoted in *Frontline*, "Transcript: In the Age of AI," PBS, November 18, 2019. www.pbs.org.

15. Shoshana Zuboff, "You Are Now Remotely Controlled," *New York Times*, January 24, 2020. www.nytimes.com.
16. Zuboff, "You Are Now Remotely Controlled."
17. Quoted in John Naughton, "'The Goal Is to Automate Us': Welcome to the Age of Surveillance Capitalism," *The Guardian* (Manchester, UK), January 20, 2019. www.theguardian.com.
18. Drew Harwell, "Giuliani Wasn't Just a Trump Partisan but a Shrewd Marketer of Vitamins, Gold, Lawsuit Says," *Washington Post*, January 26, 2021. www.washingtonpost.com.
19. Quoted in Ezra Klein, "Steve Bannon Is Onto Something," *New York Times*, January 9, 2020. www.nytimes.com.
20. Quoted in Tatum Hunter, "Surveillance Will Follow Us into 'the Metaverse,' and Our Bodies Could Be Its New Data Source," *Washington Post*, January 13, 2022. www.washingtonpost.com.
21. Quoted in Tom Huddleston Jr., "Bill Gates Says the Metaverse Will Host Most of Your Office Meetings Within 'Two or Three Years'—Here's What It Will Look Like," CNBC, December 9, 2021. www.cnbc.com.
22. Aldous Huxley, "*Brave New World* Revisited," BLTC Research, 2007. www.huxley.net.
23. Quoted in Scraps from the Loft, "*The Social Dilemma* (2020)—Transcript."

Chapter Two: Rearranging the Brain

24. Quoted in Will Conaway, "Technology Is on the Rise, While IQ Is on the Decline," *Forbes*, April 25, 2020. www.forbes.com.
25. Nicholas Carr, *The Shallows: What the Internet Is Doing to Our Brains*. New York: Norton, 2020, p. ii.
26. Joseph Firth et al., "The 'Online Brain': How the Internet May Be Changing Our Cognition," *World Psychiatry*, June 18, 2019. www.ncbi.nlm.nih.gov.
27. Quoted in ScienceDaily, "How the Internet May Be Changing the Brain," June 5, 2019. www.sciencedaily.com.
28. John Koetsier, "Digital Crack Cocaine: The Science Behind TikTok's Success," *Forbes*, January 18, 2020. www.forbes.com.
29. Quoted in Koetsier, "Digital Crack Cocaine."
30. Quoted in Koetsier, "Digital Crack Cocaine."
31. Quoted in Tim Walker, "How 'Zoom Fatigue' Impacts Communications with Students," National Education Association, October 16, 2021. www.nea.org.

32. Quoted in Walker, "How 'Zoom Fatigue' Impacts Communications with Students."
33. Brian Tait, "Understanding the Neuroscience Behind Emotional Intelligence," *Forbes*, April 22, 2020. www.forbes.com.
34. Quoted in Paul Skeldon, "Online Shopping Frustrations Impact the Brain in a Similar Way to Theft or Internet Outage," Internet Retailing, November 10, 2021. https://internetretailing.net.

Chapter Three: The Myth and Reality of Multitasking

35. Quoted in Verena von Pfetten, "Read This Story Without Distraction (Can You)," *New York Times*, April 29, 2018. www.nytimes.com.
36. Quoted in Johann Hari, "Your Attention Didn't Collapse. It Was Stolen," *The Guardian* (Manchester, UK), January 2, 2022. www.theguardian.com.
37. Quoted in Hari, "Your Attention Didn't Collapse."
38. Quoted in Johann Hari, *Stolen Focus: Why You Can't Pay Attention—and How to Think Deeply Again*. New York: Crown, 2022, p. 39.
39. Quoted in Maria Kannikova, "Multitask Masters," *New Yorker*, May 7, 2014. www.newyorker.com.
40. Quoted in Kannikova, "Multitask Masters."
41. Quoted in David Robson, "How Fraudsters Exploit Our Fears During the 'Scamdemic,'" BBC, June 13, 2021. www.bbc.com.
42. Quoted in Robson, "How Fraudsters Exploit Our Fears During the 'Scamdemic.'"
43. Quoted in Nate Schweber and Tracey Tully, "She Texted About Dinner While Driving. Then a Pedestrian Was Dead," *New York Times*, November 22, 2019. www.nytimes.com.
44. Chan Priya, "Multitasking Is a Scam: Try This Instead," Medium, December 23, 2019. https://medium.com.
45. Hari, *Stolen Focus*, pp. 40–41.
46. Quoted in Kannikova, "Multitask Masters."
47. Quoted in Hasan Al-Jarrah, "35 Multitasking Quotes on Success," Awaken the Greatness Within, 2021. www.awakenthegreatnesswithin.com.

Chapter Four: Time for a Digital Detox?

48. Kevin Roose, "Do Not Disturb: How I Ditched My Phone and Unbroke My Brain," *New York Times*, February 23, 2019. www.nytimes.com.

49. Roose, "Do Not Disturb."
50. Roose, "Do Not Disturb."
51. Roose, "Do Not Disturb."
52. Quoted in Ron Srigley, "I Asked My Students to Turn In Their Cell Phones and Write About Living Without Them," *MIT Technology Review*, December 26, 2019. www.technologyreview.com.
53. Quoted in Srigley, "I Asked My Students to Turn In Their Cell Phones and Write About Living Without Them."
54. Quoted in Srigley, "I Asked My Students to Turn In Their Cell Phones and Write About Living Without Them."
55. Arthur C. Brooks, "How to Break a Phone Addiction," *The Atlantic*, October 7, 2021. www.theatlantic.com.
56. Brooks, "How to Break a Phone Addiction."
57. Quoted in Penny Zenker, "The Productivity Toll You Need to Get a Hold of with Maths Mathisen," The Focusologist, November 6, 2020. https://pennyzenker360.com.

TIPS FOR REDUCING DIGITAL DISTRACTIONS

Digital distraction is a common problem that can interfere with learning, working, and socializing with others. These problems have attracted attention from a wide range of psychologists, researchers, and scientists who recommend the following steps for reducing the use of digital devices.

- Use an app to track online time and limit the number of launches for social media and gaming apps.
- Turn off push notifications.
- Put a rubber band around the phone to remind yourself not to pick it up.
- Schedule an hour a day for mindless scrolling.
- Delete social media and gaming apps.
- Put the phone in a different room while studying and turn it off at night.
- Get a low-tech "dumbphone" that can only be used for texts and calls.
- Take up art, music, writing, or another hobby that does not involve using a digital device.
- Participate in physical activities such as hiking, biking, and sports.

FOR FURTHER RESEARCH

Books

Goali Saedi Bocci, *The Social Media Workbook for Teens: Skills to Help You Balance Screen Time, Manage Stress, and Take Charge of Your Life*. Oakland, CA: Instant Help, 2019.

Stuart A. Kallen, *Changing Lives Through Artificial Intelligence*. San Diego, CA: ReferencePoint, 2021.

Barbara Ann Kipfer, *5,203 Things to Do Instead of Looking at Your Phone*. New York: Workman, 2020.

Erica B. Marcus, *Attention Hijacked: Using Mindfulness to Reclaim Your Brain*. Minneapolis, MN: Zest, 2022.

Alex J. Packer, *Slaying Digital Dragons*. Minneapolis, MN: Free Spirit, 2021.

Catherine Price, *How to Break Up with Your Phone*. New York: Ten Speed, 2018.

Bradley Steffens, *The Dark Side of Social Media*. San Diego, CA: ReferencePoint, 2022.

Internet Sources

Janna Anderson and Lee Rainie, "The Negatives of Digital Life," Pew Research Center, July 3, 2018. www.pewresearch.org.

Will Conaway, "Technology Is on the Rise, While IQ Is on the Decline," *Forbes*, April 25, 2020. www.forbes.com.

Kenneth Miller, "How Our Ancient Brains Are Coping in the Age of Digital Distraction," *Discover*, April 20, 2020. www.discovermagazine.com.

Hanna Schwär, "How Instagram and Facebook Are Intentionally Designed to Mimic Addictive Painkillers," Business Insider, August 11, 2021. www.businessinsider.com.

Shoshana Zuboff, "You Are Now Remotely Controlled," *New York Times*, January 24, 2020. www.nytimes.com.

Websites

Digital Wellbeing

https://wellbeing.google

Google hosts this website with numerous tips for focusing time with tech, going on a digital diet, and minimizing distractions. The site provides digital detox tools for those who use Android devices.

Information Overload Research Group

https://iorgforum.org

This organization is dedicated to helping people reduce their dependence on digital devices. The website offers solutions with blogs, videos, webinars, a YouTube channel, and podcasts.

National Day of Unplugging

www.nationaldayofunplugging.com

The National Day of Unplugging encourages people to turn off their smartphones, computers, and other digital devices for a day on the first Friday of every March. The group organizes activities in cities throughout the country and provides information about the negative effects of too much digital distraction.

Supertasker.org

https://supertasker.org

This site offers the supertasker test, which takes forty minutes and allows users to evaluate their multitasking abilities. The test is difficult, and only around 2.5 percent of test takers can expect to qualify as supertaskers.

Why We Post

www.ucl.ac.uk/why-we-post

This research project hosted by the University of London focuses on the uses and costs of social media for the global community. The site offers free online courses in multiple languages and books about the effects of social media in various countries.

INDEX

Note: Boldface page numbers indicate illustrations.

addiction and Facebook's design, 11–12
addiction to cell phones
    number of teenagers, 43
    percentage of Americans, 9
    Roose's self-treatment measures, 44–47
    Srigley's experiment, 48–49, **49**
    steps to reduce use, 50–53, **51**
adrenaline, 30
age
    cognitive decline and, 27
    of phishing targets, 37
    texting while driving and, 38
Albright, Julie, 23
alertness, brain as wired for, 5
Alphabet apps, designed to be habit forming, 10–12
American Academy of Orthopaedic Surgeons, 4
AppDetox, 52
appetite and multitasking, 39
apps
    deleting, 45
    designed to be habit forming, 10–12
    disabling notifications, 50–51
    helpful, 11
    monitoring use of, 12
    for reporting and controlling screen time, 51–53
artificial intelligence programs, 12–13, 17–18
attention economy, 8, 11

behavioral prediction, 13
blue light and sleep, 46
bottom-up stimuli, 5–6
brain
    alterations to, from excessive use of internet, 21–22
    bottom-up forces, 5–6
    cell phone use and changes in, 24–25
    complexity of, 6
    dopamine released by, 22–23
    gaming's effect on, 27, 30
    grey matter in, 27
    information overload of, 21, **22**
    MRI images of, 26
    multitasking and, 32–34
    online shopping's effects on, 29–31
    refocus time after distractions, 6
    video calls' and zooming's effects on, 26–27
brain drain, 6
Brain Imaging and Behavior, 39
Brave New World (Huxley), 18
Brooks, Arthur C., 50–51

Carnegie Mellon University, 33–34
Carr, Nicholas, 21
cell phones
    average number of daily push notifications, 53
    frequency of checking, 4
    number of teenagers addicted to, 43
    panic induced by low batteries, 5
    percentage of Americans addicted to, 9
    phishing attempts and, 36, **38**
    Screen Time feature, 44
    sleep and blue light of, 46
    usage
        annual number of days of, 52
        annual number of deaths and injuries caused by, while driving, 4
        annual number of driving accidents caused by, 4
        changes in brain and, 24–25
        communication cues missed during, 6
        daily periods free from, 50, 51
        increase in pedestrian accidents during, 4, **7**
CleverTap, 53
cognitive bias, 34–35, 37
communication, 6, 26–27
computer usage, physical effects of, 9
conspiracy entrepreneurs, 15–16
context switching, 42

deaths caused by use of cell phones while driving, 4
distractions
    average frequency of, in office, 40
    brain refocus time after, 6
    cell phone use while driving, 4, 38–39, **41**
    human appetite for, 18
    multitasking while, 37–39

paying attention to social and political situation and, 18–19
dopamine, 22–23
dumbphones, 45–46
Dunckley, Victoria L., 30

eating and multitasking, 39
education, virtual learning, 25–27
electrocardiograms, 30–31
electroencephalograms (EEGs), 29–30
emotional intelligence and gaming, 27–28
emotions while multitasking, 39, 40
Environments, 16–17
EQs (emotional quotients), 28
eye contact, 6

Facebook
    adoption of "surveillance capitalism" by, 14
    awareness of Instagram's cycle of anticipation and reward, 23
    as designed to be addictive, 10–12
    "Like" button, 8, 26
    monitoring and categorization of users, 12
Federal Bureau of Investigation, 36
fight-or-flight response
    gaming and, 30
    human evolution and, 5
    online shopping and, 31
Flipd app, 52
Flynn, James R., 20
Flynn effect, 20
FOMO (fear of missing out), 11, 18
Forest app, 52–53

gambling addiction, 23
gaming, 27, 30
Gates, Bill, 16–17
Gazzaley, Adam, 5–6, 7
gender and emotional intelligence decline, 28
Giuliani, Rudy, 15
Golumbia, David, 9–10
Gonzalez, Cleotilde, 36
Google, 10–12, 13, 14
gratification, instant, 22

Hari, Johann, 40–41
Harris, Tristan, 14, 19
Harwell, Drew, 15
Heinrich, Carolyn, 9
Hersh, Eitan, 15–16
homework and multitasking, 37
Horowitz, Evan, 21
Huxley, Aldous, 18–19

impulsivity, 27, 28

information
    intentional spreading of false, 15–16
    overloading brain with, 21, **22**
    "surveillance capitalism," 13, 14
injuries, annual number of, caused by use of cell phones while driving, 4
Instagram
    adoption of "surveillance capitalism" by, 14
    apps of, designed to be habit forming, 10–12
    cycle of anticipation and reward, 23
Instagramification, 22
intelligence
    cognitive decline and, 27
    decrease in, during twenty-first century, 20–21
    increase in, during twentieth century, 20
interference in brain, 33
internet, brain alterations from excessive use of, 21–22
IQ test, 20

Journal of Personality, 28

Koch, Christof, 6
Koetsier, John, 23

Lanier, Jaron, 12
Lewis, Jack, 31
lies, intentional spreading of, 15–16
Light Phone II, 46
"Like" button, 8, 26

magnetic resonance imaging (MRI), 26
Mansonet, Alexandra, 39
Mathisen, Maths, 52, 53
McDannald, Erin, 16
McNamee, Roger, 13
memory functions, 21
Meta, 10, 16–18, **17**
    See also Facebook; Instagram
Mezyk, Peter, 11–12
Michigan State University, 36
microexpressions, 12
Miller, Earl, 33, 34
Misra, Shalini, 6
multitasking
    avoiding pitfalls of, 39–40
    cognitive bias and, 34–35
    doing homework while, 37
    emotions while, 39, 40
    increase in eating when, 39
    in office, 40
    phishing attempts and, 36
    supertaskers when, 34–36

switch-cost and screw-up effects when, 32, 33–34, **35**
use of word, 41–42
while driving, 37–39

National Day of Unplugging, 43, 46
National Highway Traffic Safety Administration (NHTSA), 38
National Safety Council, 4
neurons and neural networks, 24
New York Times (newspaper), 44
Norris, Gareth, 37

Ohio State University, 37
online fraud, 36–37, **38**
online shopping, 28–31, **29**
overconfidence, 34–35
Oxford University (United Kingdom), 28

panic, induced by low cell phone batteries, 5
Pavlidis, Ioannis, 40
pedestrian accidents and cell phones usage, 4, **7**
Pew Research Center, 9, 43
Phelan, Hayley, 32
phishing, 36–37, **38**
"phubbing," 47
physical health and computer usage, 9
plasticity of brain, 24–25
politics, 15–16
Priya, Chan, 39–40
Proceedings of the National Academy of Sciences, 34

Qustodio, 25

Reviews.org, 4, 11, 43–44
Roose, Kevin, 44–46, 47
Rosenstein, Justin, 8–9, **10**
Rudy Giuliani's Common Sense (podcast), 15

Sarris, Jerome, 22
Sax, David, 46
scammers, 36–37, **38**
screw-up effect, 34, **35**
scrolling, 23, 50
sleep and cell phones, 46

smartphones. *See* cell phones
Social Dilemma, The (film), 14
Social Dilemma, The (Rosenstein), 8–9
social media, 5, 8–9
See also specific apps
Srigley, Ron, 48
Strayer, David, 35, 42
supertaskers, 34–36
"surveillance capitalism," 13, 14
switch-cost effect, 32, 33–34, **35**

Tait, Brian, 28
teenagers
cell phone addiction of, 43
digital diets and, 47–49, **49**
texting, 38–39, **41**
Thompson, Derek, 5
TikTok, **13**
apps of, designed to be habit forming, 10–12
as "digital crack cocaine," 23
Tinsley, Jeff, 18
Trait Emotional Intelligence Questionnaire, 28
Twitter, adoption of "surveillance capitalism" by, 14

University of California, Irvine, 6, 40–41
University of Houston, 40
University of Utah, 34

video calls and conferencing, 26–27
virtual learning, 25–27
virtual reality (VR) headsets and gloves, 16–18, **17**

Wang, Yuwen, 39
Wang, Zheng, 37
Wiederhold, Brenda, 26, 27
World Psychiatry (journal), 21

YouTube apps, 10

Zoom burnout, 26
Zoom classrooms, 26–27
Zuboff, Shoshana, 13, 14
Zuckerberg, Mark, 17

PICTURE CREDITS

Cover: Shany Muchnik/Shutterstock.com

7: Tamas-V/iStock
10: Associated Press
13: hareluya/Shutterstock.com
17: G-stock Studio/Shutterstock.com
22: Dnytro Zinkevych/Shutterstock.com
25: yurii_yurii/Shutterstock.com
29: Rawpixel.com/Shutterstock.com
35: Syda Productions/Shutterstock.com
38: mundissima/Shutterstock.com
41: Audrey_Popov/Shutterstock.com
45: Dean Drobot/Shutterstock.com
49: Monkey Business Images/Shutterstock.com
51: fizkes/Shutterstock.com

ABOUT THE AUTHOR

Stuart A. Kallen is the author of more than 350 nonfiction books for children and young adults. He has written on topics ranging from the theory of relativity to the art of electronic dance music. In 2018 Kallen won a Green Earth Book Award from the Nature Generation environmental organization for his book *Trashing the Planet: Examining the Global Garbage Glut*. In his spare time he is a singer, songwriter, and guitarist in San Diego.